The Global Health Care Chain

Routledge Research in Population & Migration

Series Editor: Paul Boyle, *University of St. Andrews*

1. Migration & Gender in the Developed World
Edited by Paul Boyle & Keith Halfacree

2. Migration, Globalisation and Human Security
Edited by David T. Graham and Nana K. Poku

3. The Geography of Trafficking and Human Smuggling
Khalid Koser and John Salt

4. Population Mobility Among Indigenous Peoples in Australasia and North America
Edited by John Taylor and Martin Bell

5. Urban Ethnic Encounters
The Spatial Consequences
Edited by Aygen Erdentug and Freek Colombijn

6. Migration in Comparative Perspective
Caribbean Communities in Britain and France
Margaret Byron and Stephanie Condon

7. Asian Migrants and European Labour Markets
Patterns and Processes of Immigrant Labour Market Insertion in Europe
Edited by Ernst Spaan, Felicitas Hillmann and Ton van Naerssen

8. Migration and Health in Asia
Edited by Santosh Jatrana, Mike Toyota and Brenda S.A. Yeoh

9. Retirement Migration
Paradoxes of Ageing
Caroline Oliver

10. The International Migration of Health Workers
Edited by John Connell

11. Refugees, Recent Migrants and Employment
Challenging Barriers and Exploring Pathways
Edited by Sonia McKay

12. The Global Health Care Chain
From the Pacific to the World
John Connell

The Global Health Care Chain

From the Pacific to the World

John Connell

Routledge
Taylor & Francis Group
LONDON AND NEW YORK

Published 2009
by Routledge
2 Park Square, Milton Park, Abingdon, Oxon OX14 4RN

Simultaneously published in the UK
by Routledge
52 Vanderbilt Avenue, New York, NY 10017

Routledge is an imprint of the Taylor & Francis Group, an informa business

First issued in paperback 2012

Typeset in Sabon by IBT Global.

Library of Congress Cataloging in Publication Data

Connell, John, 1946–
The global health care chain : from the Pacific to the world / by John Connell.
p. ; cm. — (Routledge research in population & migration ; 12)
Includes bibliographical references and index.
1. Medical personnel—Pacific Area. 2. Emigration and immigration—Pacific Area. I. Title. II. Series: Routledge research in population and migration ; 12.

[DNLM: 1. Health Personnel—Pacific Islands. 2. Developing Countries—Pacific Islands. 3. Emigration and Immigration—Pacific Islands. 4. Health Manpower—Pacific Islands. 5. Transients and Migrants—Pacific Islands. W 21 C752g 2009]
RA410.9.P16C66 2009
362.1—dc22
2008033863

ISBN 13: 978-0-415-54318-7 (pbk)
ISBN13: 978-0-415-95622-2 (hbk)
ISBN13: 978-0-203-88511-6 (ebk)

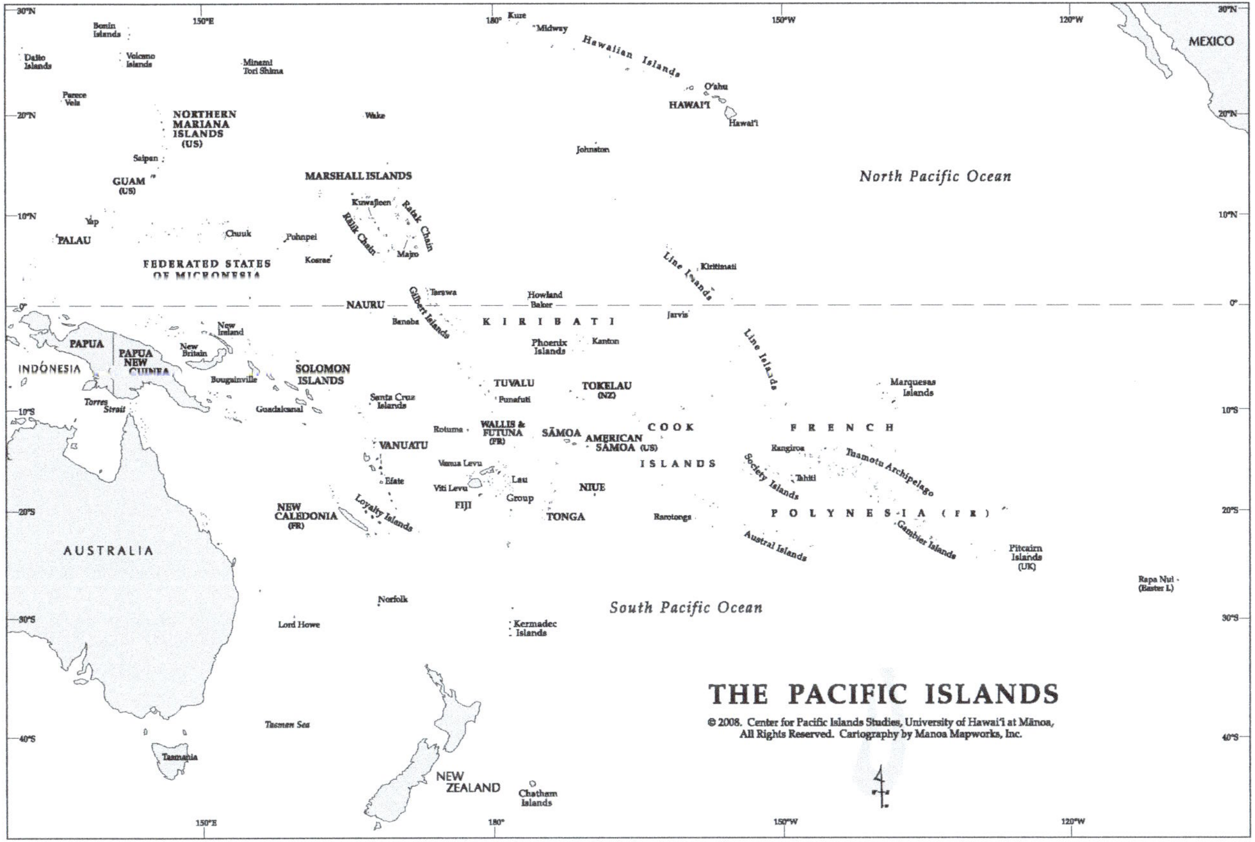
THE PACIFIC ISLANDS
© 2008. Center for Pacific Islands Studies, University of Hawai'i at Mānoa,
All Rights Reserved. Cartography by Manoa Mapworks, Inc.
North Pacific Ocean
South Pacific Ocean
MEXICO
Hawaiian Islands
Kure
Midway
O'ahu
HAWAI'I
Hawai'i
Johnston
Wake
Bonin Islands
Volcano Islands
Minami Tori Shima
Daito Islands
Parece Vela
NORTHERN MARIANA ISLANDS (US)
Saipan
GUAM (US)
MARSHALL ISLANDS
Kwajalein
Ratak Chain
Ralik Chain
Majro
Yap
PALAU
Chuuk
Pohnpei
Kosrae
FEDERATED STATES OF MICRONESIA
NAURU
Tarawa
Gilbert Islands
Banaba
Howland
Baker
K I R I B A T I
Phoenix Islands
Kanton
Line Islands
Kiritimati
Jarvis
PAPUA
PAPUA NEW GUINEA
INDONESIA
New Ireland
New Britain
Bougainville
SOLOMON ISLANDS
Guadalcanal
Torres Strait
Santa Cruz Islands
TUVALU
Funafuti
TOKELAU (NZ)
Rotuma
WALLIS & FUTUNA (FR)
SĀMOA
AMERICAN SAMOA (US)
COOK ISLANDS
VANUATU
Efate
Vanua Levu
Viti Levu
FIJI
Lau Group
NIUE
TONGA
Rarotonga
NEW CALEDONIA (FR)
Loyalty Islands
Marquesas Islands
FRENCH POLYNESIA (FR)
Rangiroa
Tuamotu Archipelago
Tahiti
Society Islands
Gambier Islands
Austral Islands
Pitcairn Islands (UK)
Rapa Nui (Easter I.)
AUSTRALIA
Norfolk
Lord Howe
Kermadec Islands
Tasman Sea
Tasmania
NEW ZEALAND
Chatham Islands
30°N
20°N
10°N
0°
10°S
20°S
30°S
40°S
150°E
180°
150°W
120°W

For Thantida, with love

'Nurse' The Changes

Then,
it was a coveted profession,
the dream vocation
of the daughters of Samoa.
It was then,
that you dared to idolize
selfless humanity,
care giving to the suffering
the only touch of human compassion
in the regimented atmosphere
of starched white discipline
and corridors of eroded emotions.
It was then
that you imagined,
pride fluttering in white caps,
motivation forever scurrying
yet never heard above
the footfalls of white plastic,
warmth flowing from ice cold machines
and monotonous IVs.
Today,
it is just another eight hour daily ritual
sought after by the job hungry youth
some without a vision for the call.
Yet today she is still the expected lighter 'of the lamp'
and be the gatekeeper
to keep the vigil and perform miracles
where the government purse
has not been suitably strung
to attract even the shadow
of a doctor.
Today, she is pulled

by the demands of extra skills
to meet an ever changing role,
her sights set on the elevation of academia
for recognition of a rightful place
in a world of changing policies
and cost cutting technology.
Take leaps where there are no bounds.
Run with the rush of the tide.
Seek due praise of your profession.
Sing out that you are not an endangered species
BUT, sing it still with a human voice

Noumea Simi
(Apia, Samoa)

Reprinted with permission of Allen and Unwin from Barclay, L, Fenwick, J, Nielson, F, Poston-Sanderson, B, Stowers, P and Wilkinson, J (1998) *Samoan Nursing.*

Contents

Abbreviations

ADB	Asian Development Bank
ASEAN	Association of South-East Asian Nations
CFA	Compact of Free Association
CMI	College of the Marshall Islands
EU	European Union
FNA	Fiji Nursing Association
FSM	Federated States of Micronesia
FScM	Fiji School of Medicine
GDP	Gross Domestic Product
HDI	Human Development Index
HIV/AIDS	Human Immunodeficiency Virus/Acquired Immune Deficiency Syndrome
ICU	Intensive Care Unit
IMR	Infant Mortality Rate
IT	Information Technology
MDGs	Millennium Development Goals
MIRAB	Migration—Remittances—Aid—Bureaucracy
MOH	Ministry of Health
NCDs	Non-Communicable Diseases
NGO	Non-Governmental Organization
PHC	Primary Health Care
PNG	Papua New Guinea
SHW	Skilled Health Worker
TTPI	Trust Territory of the Pacific Islands
UAE	United Arab Emirates
UNV	United Nations Volunteers
URT	Upper Respiratory Tract Infection
USP	University of the South Pacific
WHO	World Health Organization

Preface

In recent years there has been a substantial increase in skilled migration, not only of health workers. This reflects the growth and internationalization of the service sector and rising demand for skilled workers in developed countries (where training is relatively costly). Increasingly migration is determined by skill status. The health sector is rather different from other skilled sectors since most employment is in the public sector, where conditions have tended to worsen (relatively and sometimes absolutely) with restructuring; technology cannot replace workers and the rise of HIV/AIDS and the aging of populations have put new demands on a sometimes diminishing health workforce. At the same time there is now a greater range of jobs for women, beyond a sector that is now seen by some as dirty and dangerous (and unrewarding). Restructuring, often externally imposed, has similarly affected health systems in developing countries, contributing to concerns over wages, working conditions, training and other issues, all of which have stimulated new forms of international migration, linking both developing and developed countries into what has become a global care chain.

Although there have been various accounts of the migration of skilled health workers in several parts of the world, a sample of which are in the companion volume (*The International Migration of Health Workers*), this book seeks to provide a more thorough and detailed analysis of this growing phenomenon in a part of the world where it has recently become significant, so much so that the Pacific island nations have collectively sought to develop a Code of Practice to mitigate the impacts of overseas migration and recruitment. International migration of skilled health workers has gone on for over a quarter of a century, but in the last decade with critical changes in both sending and receiving countries, most parts of the Pacific are now significantly affected by the consequences of this migration. Here, as elsewhere, it has become a controversial issue.

Much of the book is based on a survey undertaken in the Pacific, of more than five hundred workers in nine island states and three destination states—Australia, Canada and New Zealand. The book therefore seeks to take the understanding of health worker migration substantially beyond the more scattered and fragmented papers and anecdotes that largely existed before, towards a more consolidated analysis. In doing so it reveals the exceptional significance of migration for both sending and receiving countries, and casts new light on gender, globalization, transnational linkages, remittances, the trade in services and the critical relationship between migration and development. Despite the large sample the book largely avoids quantitative analysis, which would have given a somewhat spurious accuracy to complex social contexts, in favour of a perhaps unduly fragmented 'ethnography'.

The book focuses on nine Pacific island countries, in three subtly different cultural regions—Micronesia (Kiribati, Marshall Islands and Palau), Melanesia (Fiji and Vanuatu) and Polynesia (Cook Islands, Niue, Samoa and Tonga). It also makes passing reference to other Pacific island states where similar contexts exist. All islanders are referred to here as living in states, though some smaller 'states' have no effective independent political status but are overseas territories of metropolitan states. The people of the region have either been referred to according to their national status or as Pacific islanders, an inadequate term for the vast diversity of the region but one that has not been superseded. Those of Indian descent in Fiji are referred to as Indo-Fijians, though other terms have sometimes been preferred elsewhere.

I am grateful to a number of people in several countries for assistance with the data collection, and especially the conducting of questionnaire surveys. These include, in the Cook Islands, Kiribati and the Marshall Islands, Hazel Easthope; in Fiji, Taiamoni Tongamoa; in Samoa, Tautala'aso Taulealo and Keneti Vaigafa; in Tonga, Nicole Maron and Taiamoni Tongamoa; in Vanuatu, Vivien Dunne and Sarah Naupa; in Palau, Julie Tellei (on behalf of the Palau Resource Institute); in Niue, Bob Talagi; in Canada, Charles Greenberg; in New Zealand, Sitaleki Finau; and in Australia, Carmen Voigt-Graf and Paulina Fusitu'a. I am particularly grateful to Lorraine Kerse, formerly of WHO, for her continuous support for this project, and to WHO for funding the early phases of the work. I must again thank Ben Holtzman of Routledge for his customary patience, Lorraine Kerse and Richard Taylor for reading various chapters and Monica Liem for sorting out my wayward formatting. Ultimately I am most indebted to the many nurses, doctors and other health workers who gave their very valuable time to participate in the survey and to the Ministries and Departments of Health in the various countries who made this possible. Comments have rarely been attributed to particular individuals, and have been made as anonymous as possible, to ensure confidentiality. All quotations, unless otherwise stated, are from skilled health workers in the Pacific islands or in migrant destinations.

John Connell,
School of Geosciences, University of Sydney.
May 2008

1 The Globalization of Skilled Migration

A Pacific Perspective

> Islands that are so renowned for the quality of their nursing professionals end up losing them for that very reason: their quiet and humble efficiency that proves to be such great value for money in the bigger paramedical markets of the developed world. Every year nurses who have trained in the Pacific islands and earned their spurs there, leave for greener pastures, literally in droves. It's exactly like the way most islands lose their finest sportspersons to their metropolitan neighbours—often fighting against their own home teams for their employers.
>
> (*Islands Business*, July 2007)

Migration of skilled health workers (SHWs) within, into but especially from Pacific island states is widely considered to be a growing problem. It is certainly growing in significance, alongside the migration of many others, in what has become in this century something of an outward urge. Waves of increasingly diverse migration characterize the contemporary Pacific. The costly emigration of scarce and expensively trained human capital affects core national strategies for health sector development. Training of SHWs is particularly expensive because of the long duration, the high costs of teaching materials and techniques (and the need for post-graduate education and training programmes) which must be set against the limited resources of small island states. Replacements can also be costly (and may lack appropriate skills, languages and cultural sensitivity) whilst ensuring their adequacy is difficult. Why these migrations occur and their impact on satisfying basic needs, achieving sustainable health strategies and developing healthy islands are the issues at the core of this book.

The migration of Pacific SHWs is no new phenomenon. At least as early as 1989 a medical degree from the Fiji School of Medicine was regarded by some as a 'passport to prosperity'. However, until quite recently, there have been few studies of any facet of this migration, though the media at least have drawn attention to what they see as excessive migration through a series of dramatic headlines such as 'Nurses set to leave in droves' (*Fiji Times*, 12 February 2003), 'Nurse exodus" (*Sunday Post* [Fiji], 23 March 2003) and 'Nurse crisis hits rural centre' (*Fiji Times*, 28 March 2003). While these headlines are from one particular year in Fiji they can be replicated across the region for much of the present century. Cartoons (Figure 1.1)

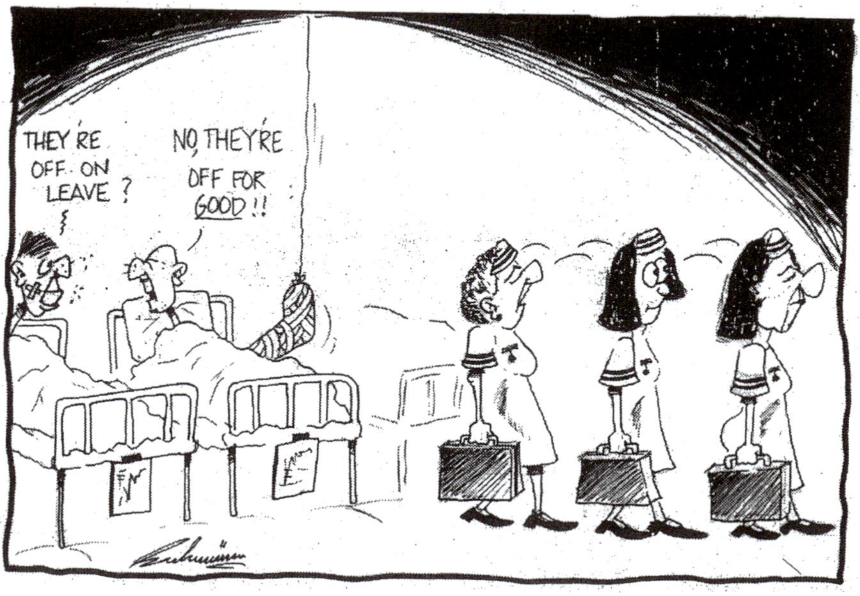
THEY'RE OFF ON LEAVE ?
NO, THEY'RE OFF FOR GOOD !!

Figure 1.1 On the move?
Credit: *Fiji Times*, 12 February 2003

provide even more dramatic impact. Few studies in the Pacific region have otherwise examined skilled migration (cf. Liki 1994, 2001; Voigt-Graf 2003; Voigt-Graf, Iredale and Khoo 2007). There are remarkably few studies in the Pacific island states of the migration of skilled workers.

Human capital is critical for the economic and social development of all societies, and health is a universal basic need. In the health arena the significance of human resources is doubled. Health workers directly improve the quality of life for others, who can then contribute more to wider society. Conversely, a lack of health workers has harmful ramifications for the rest of society, most evident in developing countries where needs are considerable. Some categories of health workers, especially nurses, are in particular global demand, while migration has been most evident for a number of sub-Saharan African countries, and also for small island states in the Caribbean and the Pacific, constituting part of a general movement from the more impoverished south to the wealthier north. Unsurprisingly, this migration from relatively poor to relatively rich countries has been a source of global concern (Connell 2008c), especially as that migration has become more global, complex and hierarchical and so more challenging to poorer states, where wages and working conditions are usually least adequate. It has been a critical influence on the ability of countries to manage human resources and therefore health service delivery.

The accelerated global migration of SHWs has gradually involved most Pacific island states, but with migration mainly to the metropolitan states on the Pacific Rim. Skilled migration has occurred in a much wider cultural and migration context, part of the creation of household 'transnational corporations of kin' involving extended households, with great significance for the flow of remittances to island microstates where economic growth is weak or non-existent. Migration, substantial in Polynesia for half a century, has responded to widespread perceptions of relative deprivation with respect to the Pacific Rim. This has resulted in the movement of workers away from health services which face considerable challenges, because of the fragmentation of island states, low budgets devoted to health care, the associated rise of non-communicable diseases (NCDs) and the emergence of HIV/AIDS (Chapter 2).

Pacific migration is part of a situation where, in just the last few years, international migration has become of extraordinary global significance, especially in Europe, with changes in the shape and structure of the European Union (EU). This has necessitated considerable rethinking of the role of migration, and especially of the 'brain drain'. In the context of health, numerous studies, mainly in Africa, have examined the impact of this, and made recommendations on new policy formation, such as fair codes of recruitment and compensatory mechanisms, though little has actually changed. So-called 'knowledge workers', notably health workers and those in information technology (IT), experience greater mobility compared with most service workers. Skilled migration has increasingly involved independent networks that disregard national boundaries, despite parallel attempts to strengthen borders against unskilled and refugee migration. Nation-states have been unable to respond with vision and imagination to the challenges posed by rising levels of migration, and especially the fluidity and immediacy of skilled migration, embodied in new notions of transnationalism, and multinational social networks.

Increased migration of skilled workers is a response to the accelerated globalization of the service sector. Such professional services as health care are very much part of this new internationalization of labour, seemingly paradoxically because of relatively low wages and poor working conditions in the destination countries (e.g. Gish and Godfrey 1979; Buchan and O'May 2000; Hardill and MacDonald 2000; Raghuram and Kofman 2002). In many metropolitan states jobs in the health sector are seen as too demanding and poorly paid, while demand has increased with the aging of developed country populations. Greater longevity, more chronic diseases and rising expectations of health and health care have increased demands for care and on care workers. Wages have fallen behind increases in the cost of living, and employment in the public sector (not only in health) is no longer favourably perceived. Relative declines in public sector funding have enhanced that perception. Many developed countries, including Australia, the United States and New Zealand, the main destinations of

Pacific SHWs, have a particular shortage of nurses, especially in remote areas. This has followed high attrition rates and low recruitment, resulting from dislike of shift-work, lack of flexibility, poor work conditions and incomes, while family responsibilities have resulted in the choice of a job more suited to flexible lifestyles. Reduced recruitment of health workers has followed declining birth-rates, hence there are fewer younger people, and more diverse employment opportunities for women, many of which offer superior wages and working conditions, alongside greater prestige and respect.

Ironically, problems of recruitment and attrition in developed countries are similar to the reasons that SHWs in the Pacific have left their own national health services. They have migrated for financial reasons, social reasons (including further education for themselves and other family members overseas) and professional concerns over the inadequacy of the local health sector in terms of the broad conditions of employment (Chapter 5). Migration occurs because it provides higher incomes, and thus better living conditions for migrants and their families, alongside new experiences and the acquisition of superior professional expertise while migrant remittances enhance the lives of the kin who remain at home.

THE GLOBAL CARE CHAIN

The international migration of SHWs has gone through three broad phases, increasingly involving more people and places. Not only has there been recognition of a global health care chain, but migration has been seen as involving 'stepping stones' in a 'carousel of complexity' as SHWs engage in 'cascade migration'—what was once more simply step migration—moving between countries and increasingly through a series of stages where, for many, the ultimate goal is the United States, where the grass is assuredly greenest. Such a flurry of new metaphors and analogies depict the significance of an increasingly global migration system.

International migration of SHWs was ignored until the 1960s. But earlier migration constituted a first phase, largely the movement of health workers from western nations to their colonies, often in association with missionary endeavours. Health was poor and mortality rates high, especially in the tropics, diseases such as leprosy and malaria were common and, although health care was officially a priority in many colonies, in the Pacific resources were thinly spread, the administration was primarily concerned with the welfare of labour recruits and mission activities were therefore invaluable (Lambert 1941; Maddocks 1975). As in large parts of Africa, missions were often the only source of nursing care, most hospitals had been built by them and missionaries usually received some medical training (Firth 1997; Rubinstein 1999). In large parts of the Pacific the relationship between the missions and health services was extremely close, at least until independence in the 1970s and 1980s when government services became dominant. In Papua New Guinea (PNG) refugee doctors from Hungary, Poland, Ukraine and elsewhere (whose qualifications were not recognised in Australia) were a substantial cohort of the post-war intake of doctors, and subsequently doctors came from Britain and Australia (Denoon 1989: 74). Similar situations characterized most of the Pacific. Throughout much of Melanesia health services outside the main towns remain routinely linked to missions. In its colonial phase the movement of these pioneer health workers was entirely from places with relatively good health to those where health care was greatly needed.

Almost half a century ago, the direction of migration shifted, as the first movements began from a few developing countries to a small number of developed countries, typified by the recruitment of nurses from the Philippines for the Middle East (Mejia, Pizurki and Royston 1979). Larger independent developing countries, such as India, Pakistan and Iran, were the sources of thousands of SHWs, mainly doctors, for western countries such as Britain, Australia, Canada and particularly the United States. This second phase was the start of what quickly became recognised as a brain drain, a term first applied in the 1970s to the movement of scientists, doctors and other highly qualified people (Gish 1971). This phase had no relevance in Pacific states with so few SHWs.

After something of a hiatus, migration has now extended, in a third phase, to become more complex, more globally comprehensive (with the new significance of sub-Saharan Africa), increasingly involving governments and recruiting agencies, and dominated by women, as the core occupations have shifted from medicine to nursing. New movements of nurses into and between relatively developed countries, and the recent entries of China as a source and Japan as a recipient of nurses, characterize this gendered and global flow. Until recently it has tended to follow post-colonial, and thus language, ties but has gradually become much more diverse, posing some linguistic complexities.

This third phase is of particular significance for the Pacific. While the United States, Canada and much of western Europe intensified their needs for migrant health workers, Australia and New Zealand too became major recipients of overseas health workers (beyond their traditional European sources of supply). Thus the four Anglophone metropolitan countries on the fringes of the Pacific became global destinations. While most drew health workers from Asia, especially the Philippines, each became destinations for Pacific SHWs, as they already were for other migrants from the region.

The Pacific region has thus been drawn into a context where international recruitment of nurses has become increasingly global. There are now new movements of nurses between relatively developed countries, for example from South Africa and Finland to the United Kingdom. Ireland, once an exporter, is now an active recruiter (Yeates 2008). Something of a hierarchy characterizes the global migration chain from impoverished

Asian states and the relatively small and poor island states of the Caribbean and Pacific, to the developed world. A growing number of countries, including Finland and the Philippines, deliberately produce excess numbers of nurses to supply overseas markets. The greater complexity of migration is evident in the interlocking chains of recruitment and supply, some of which were in place thirty years ago (Mejia, Pizurki and Royston 1979). Thus Australia and New Zealand recruit and absorb from the Pacific island states (which recruit from Burma and China) as they in turn supply the United Kingdom. Fiji loses nurses to the Marshall Islands and Palau; many move on to the United States, the United Kingdom and the United Arab Emirates (UAE). In the Caribbean, Guyanan nurses move to several countries, including St. Lucia and Jamaica. Jamaican nurses travel to the Virgin Islands and the United States, while Jamaica recruits from Ghana (Connell 2007e). Dependent territories, such as Anguilla in the Caribbean and Guam and American Samoa in the Pacific, gain workers from nearby independent states. In both the Caribbean and the Pacific, two-tier systems, part of the hierarchy within the global care chain, link relatively small and poor island states to nearby richer states and territories, and then onwards to the developed world, culminating in the United States. As demand in developed countries has increased, the structure of recruitment has grown and extended. Many countries are both sending and receiving countries—particularly such large states as the United Kingdom and Australia, but also smaller states such as Barbados and Fiji (van Eyck 2004). There is now even competition between island states, involving recruitment by three Micronesian states (Federated States of Micronesia, Marshall Islands and Palau) from Fiji, alongside recruitment from New Zealand and Gulf States such as the UAE. Migration is constantly in flux depending on market demands, domestic pressures, new forms of global legislation and codes of practice, and perceptions of amenable and profitable destinations.

Most Pacific island states, like developing countries elsewhere, experience shortages of workers, which leave gaps in the public and sometimes private sectors. Overall shortages tend to be aggravated by uneven distribution within countries, the movement of health workers from rural to urban areas, and from the public to the private sector, alongside attrition and retirement. As demand in rich countries increases, such shortages are likely to persist, and unless there is greater recruitment into the health workforce, less attrition or significant policy change elsewhere, migration too is likely to continue. Changing expectations will place further demands on health systems.

Globalization of the migration of SHWs, simply defined as those who have undergone more than a year's tertiary training in the health sector, poses new costs for supplying nations, that generally amount to domestic shortages and therefore unmet health needs, and increased inequity in access to health care (Chapter 6). If migration is very substantial, as in several sub-Saharan African countries, where the majority of medical school graduates migrate to developed countries and health needs are great, the costs are considerable (Connell et al. 2007). This international transfer of human resources unequivocally takes SHWs from areas of high need and demand to their converse. The third phase of international migration thus amplified the second in its increasing orientation towards developed countries, the extension of sources to newer nations and the increasing involvement of women. High proportions of skilled emigrants exemplify several Pacific states; about half of all Samoa and Tonga's doctors and a quarter of Fiji and Solomon Islands' doctors work overseas, to the extent that certain specialized facilities have closed because of the lack of skilled workers, and other costs are evident (Chapter 6). Critical development issues accompany the migration of SHWs.

SMALL ISLAND STATES

Human resource management and development planning are particularly difficult in small island states; although needs are no fewer, the real and potential supply of skilled workers is limited. Employment within small states holds particular problems absent from larger ones. The size of the public sector workforce may be disproportionately high, since a minimum number of functions and workers are crucial. (In the Pacific, notably in Micronesia, some small states inherited bloated colonial bureaucracies with limited relationship to local needs). Migration can take a substantial toll on workforces, especially where very small numbers of workers with distinct skills, such as radiologists or anæsthetists, are required, and local training facilities are absent, further complicating human resource planning and forecasting.

Relatively small numbers of skilled workers are often concentrated in the centre, especially since most island states experience a high degree of urban primacy, with just one real urban centre. Only the larger states of PNG and Fiji have an urban hierarchy more typical of developed countries. Consequently the urban concentration of skilled workers is accentuated by urban bias, with development expenditure highly concentrated at the centre and rural and regional facilities often inadequate. Obvious economies of scale may translate into a simple neglect of outlying areas where the costs of service delivery are great and cultural minorities more likely to be present. Decentralization similarly proves difficult when there is little to decentralize, and fragmentation adds additional costs. In the health sector this has tended to emphasize the 'inverse care law', where facilities are most evident and effective where they are least needed.

Retention of skilled workers may be particularly difficult in small states, with centralized bureaucracies where many public servants know each other well, hence the task of developing merit-based recruitment and promotion is extremely difficult, even when and where the intent exists. Where there have been losses of skills, 'the brain drain has been one reason for the promotion of inadequate people' (Jacobs 1975: 142), as the more adequate leave either in frustration or in search of superior opportunities. This may be accentuated by social divisions, significant in most Pacific states, based on ethnicity, language or place of origin. Similarly, being in some form of opposition, even within a hospital management context, where elite structures converge and many roles are played by the same individual, may be grim and lead to 'institutional death and/or emigration' (Baldacchino 1997: 75). Even without such tensions, the smaller the administration, the fewer the possibilities for a lifetime career within it simply because of the reduced number of promotion opportunities towards the top, which in itself creates frustration, especially if transparent, merit-based promotion is lacking. Numbers are few, anonymity is almost impossible; relationships are more intense, necessitating careful management. Individuals are more likely to hold the monopoly on certain scarce and valued jobs; newly trained and hired workers find a variety of ceilings to promotion and innovations percolate slowly. Yet small administrations tend to have very limited spare capacity so that the absence of any worker, whether because of training, sickness, leave or migration, places disproportionate pressure on those who remain.

Rather differently the absence of economies of scale works 'in reverse' in small states, both because skilled workers are drawn from limited pools of people and because, where certain items of expenditure occur in large discrete amounts, there can be a choice between either excess capacity or going without (May and Tupouniua 1980: 428), a situation which affects the provision of infrastructure, supplies and also human resources. In most small states, and certainly those in the Pacific, the small size of countries, the dominant role of the government, limited urbanization and personal wealth have discouraged the private sector from significant involvement in the economy, let alone traditional public spheres such as health, resulting in repeated invocations from external agencies for enhanced private sector development (e.g. Asian Development Bank [ADB] 2004). The dominance of the public sector gives limited room to manoeuvre in terms of employment for most citizens and it may be that 'the alert and ambitious become adept at protecting themselves from, or even better ingratiating themselves with, politicians and civil servants' (Baldacchino 1997: 70), which minimizes employment flexibility and blocks initiatives.

Such problems are absorbed in other constraints to development; hence, 'it is not always easy to disentangle the effects of smallness from those of remoteness and peripheralness' (Davies 1985: 248). A litany of problems face island microstates, both internal, from limited resources, populations (and thus markets and a skilled workforce), and external, as they face the whims and uncertainties of natural disasters, commodity price fluctuations, aid donors, transnational corporations and tour operators, most of which island states have little capacity to influence, other than through moral precepts, as is evident in current debates on climate change, and also over codes of practice for migration (Chapter 7). Island states are characterized by an unusual degree of vulnerability to natural and human-induced phenomena.

Set against these disadvantages, island states have few obvious advantages; isolation has led to a degree of cultural integrity, and sometimes escape from the ravages of environmental degradation, but the distance that may once have lent enchantment for external observers is now a brake on various features of modern development, creating high costs for imported goods from oil to medical technology, and from pharmaceuticals to foods. Small island states generally, and more isolated and fragmented Pacific states in particular, face inherent development problems centred around their human resources that are greater than those in most larger states, and are often compounded by the practice of development.

THE PACIFIC ISLANDS AND HEALTH CARE RESOURCES

The more than twenty Pacific island states are scattered across an ocean that covers a third of the earth's surface, and have a combined population of little more than nine million, more than two thirds of whom are in PNG. An area of exceptional geographical, cultural and economic diversity is further complicated by fragmentation, restricted land areas, weak infrastructures and isolation. Most Pacific island states have numerous populated islands and, in Melanesia, many distinct languages and cultural groups. Many islands are isolated, even within countries, economies are poorly linked to the wider world and services are fragmentary beyond the few significant urban centres. Isolation has meant that indigenous cultures, at least in Melanesia, have been relatively unchanged and semi-subsistence economies typify parts of the region. The prospects for sustained economic development are poor compared with many other regions of the world and in the 1990s some of the difficulties attached to social and economic development have been reflected in political crises in some states. There are now widely perceived differences in economic growth and social welfare between the island states and those of the metropolitan fringe, hence the consequent substantial and accelerated migration to the Pacific Rim.

Health systems in most island states experienced significant attrition and migration rates during the 1990s and early 2000s, accompanying the widespread down-sizing (or stabilizing) of public service numbers. This followed minimal economic growth and growing external pressures on island states to engage in comprehensive restructuring. Nonetheless, the situation was already of concern:

> The region faces a crisis in terms of its health work force, not only in terms of direct care providers but at all levels of the system. It is not surprising that one of the most frequently mentioned topics is the shortage

> of doctors. . .. The physician shortage is only the tip of the iceberg . . . Inefficiency in health systems is a major problem and there is a crucial need for trained administrative personnel. (Lewis 1990: 84)

The human resource situation is sometimes most acute in the smaller states of the region, partly because of the small numbers involved. One dramatic example of this was the observation in a report by a Pacific island (Kiribati) doctor that a new doctor would soon arrive in the very small island state of Tokelau in 2000; hence, prior to that there was 'a need to create a good incentive package to prevent this new doctor from leaving to neighbouring countries' (Taitai 1999: 39). Presumptions of future migration are well founded and well entrenched. It is in this apparently worsening context that the present study is situated.

Some measure of the significance of migration and its context is evident from the meeting of the South Pacific Nurses Forum in August 2002. The conference summary statement is indicative of the range of concerns from nurses alone.

> The shortage of nurses and midwives across the South Pacific was discussed and countries shared some of their strategies to recruit and retrain nurses. New Zealand spoke about pre-entry programs and pathways to registered nurses training. Australia shared their experience with re-entry and refresher programs and said that the cost of such programs was a barrier and that scholarships were being offered so that nurses could access the programs. Fiji advised that they were encouraging some of their older nurses to come out of retirement and work for a further five years (i.e. from age 55 to age 60). Nurses from the smaller Pacific countries were attracted to work in New Zealand and Australia where the salary remuneration was better. Most countries felt that more people needed to be recruited into nursing courses, particularly young people and that working conditions for nurses and salary levels needed to be improved to encourage nurses to stay in the workforce. The issue of countries poaching each others' nurses was also raised. While the ability to gain education and experience in other countries was seen as a benefit of nursing, SPNF countries expressed concern at the recruitment of local nurses by other countries. (South Pacific Nurses Forum 2002: 4)

The Forum concluded by endorsing the International Council of Nurses Position Statement on Ethical Recruitment that sought to establish mechanisms for reciprocity and the discontinuation of migration from the most affected states (Chapter 7). Subsequent meetings of Pacific Health Ministers have raised similar issues, developed similar themes, supported a regional code of practice and sought to reduce problematic migration.

All the issues that affect health systems and health workers are a function of other related problems in Pacific island states (and island states more generally): shortages of financial resources, inadequate government commitment to health in several states (despite the linkage between poor health and slower economic growth), weak management capacity, few economies of scale (that contribute to shortages of drugs and technology, alongside human resources). This is also linked to a dependence on overseas facilities (such as education and training facilities and specialist hospitals), alongside rising expectations for the delivery of services and standards of living. In some places this has led to an emphasis on advanced technology (and on hospitals) rather than on appropriate technology, preventative health care and the achievement of a balanced workforce. In many states there are weaknesses in governance and political will (involving organization and commitment at all levels), a lack of interest in the health sector as a place of employment and, more generally, the lack of a 'stakeholder society'. An underlying problem in many states is simply a lack of capital. Consequently there are a range of both long-standing and relatively new constraints to developing a more responsive and appropriate health care system.

THE STUDY

Evidence of shortages of SHWs has accumulated in recent years. The last detailed overview of the health workforce stock in the Pacific was undertaken in 1990 (Rotem and Dewdney 1991), covering twelve island states. It excluded some of those (Marshall Islands, Niue and Tuvalu) where migration was perceived to be a problem, but showed that there were already problems relating to the retention of SHWs in several states (e.g. Federated States of Micronesia [FSM], Fiji, Palau, Tonga and Samoa), alongside shortages of skilled workers in certain areas. Both Fiji and Samoa then referred specifically to an existing brain drain, whilst both Palau and Samoa experienced high attrition rates for their overseas trained health workers (few of whom returned). Since then migration has accelerated, both in numbers and in the proportion of the skilled health workforce that this represents. Most countries have had to rely on donor support and direct recruitment to compensate for the loss of health workers; other countries have kept SHWs in service past retirement age. In some other contexts, where there has been a substantial emigration of SHWs, as in India (and perhaps in the Philippines), there has been some argument that this does not constitute a brain or skill drain, but is actually an overflow (Oommen 1989) in the sense that national needs are presently satisfied, but this is not the situation in the Pacific.

Previous studies of the migration of SHWs have made various observations concerning the effect of migration on health care, though there is often little solid empirical data to support these observations. They include the basic loss of health skills (on the assumption that lost skills must necessarily result in worsened health care outcomes), especially in rural and remote areas; the reduced morale and greater workload of those who remain; the immigration of replacements (who may not have appropriate qualifications, or may lack the language, commitment and cultural sensitivity to deal with local issues); the cost of referrals (both domestically and internationally) where local expertise is unavailable. Overall these suggest that health services have experienced reduced efficiency (e.g. delays in receiving acute emergency care and long waiting times for scheduled services), and may have become more costly, with some reduction in equity of access to basic health services. None of these effects have been examined closely or systematically in the Pacific, and there may be compensating tendencies (e.g. the aid-financed delivery of specialized heart and ophthalmological services in some states) though these cannot be depended on for continuity, and do not contribute to long-term sustainable health care.

The study on which this book is based was designed to develop these conclusions further through an interlocking series of surveys of movers, stayers and returnees, which primarily focused on doctors (Medical Officers) and graduate nurses, and to a lesser extent other SHWs in less numerous occupational groups. The study was undertaken between 2000 and 2005 in nine Pacific island states: including four in Polynesia (Samoa, Tonga, Niue and the Cook Islands), three in Micronesia (Kiribati, Marshall Islands and Palau) and two in Melanesia (Fiji and Vanuatu) and in two key destinations: Sydney (Australia) and Auckland (New Zealand). It sought to provide a cross-section across larger and smaller states in the region, and across the three cultural areas, but largely ignored those countries that have retained close political ties to metropolitan states, particularly the French and American territories, where human and financial resources have tended to be more substantial. The surveys focused on migration histories, attitudes to the health profession and the propensity to migrate. Initially these were undertaken in the capital cities, but were later extended to smaller urban centres and more remote islands, and supplemented by some extended conversations. In the smaller towns and outer islands it was generally evident that pressures on health workers, and the propensity to migrate, were somewhat greater, and demand for adequate health care was less likely to be satisfied. The final element of the study focused on the immigration of doctors and nurses into the Pacific; this concentrated on Cook Islands, Kiribati, Marshall Islands, Fiji, Palau and Vanuatu, where numbers were relatively high. Over 470 questionnaires were completed within the island states, proportionally more in the larger countries—Fiji (over a hundred) and Samoa, and fewest in Niue (25), and a further seventy outside, these being mainly undertaken by snowball sampling. More than two-thirds of the sample were nurses, and relatively few had 'other' skills, while more than 95 percent of the nurses were women, and about two-thirds of the doctors were men, all a reflection of the structure of the health sector.

2 The Pacific Islands and Health Care

The Pacific island region, as conventionally defined, includes almost a thousand language and cultural groups and over three hundred populated islands. The larger Melanesian states in the west can loosely be characterized by internal migration, the Polynesian states to the east by extensive international migration and the smaller Micronesian states to the north by both internal and increasingly international migration. The most substantial emigration streams in the region have come from the central Polynesian states (Tonga, Samoa, Niue, the Cook Islands and Tokelau), Fiji and, increasingly, the Micronesian states of Palau, the Marshall Islands and the FSM. Health status is best in those states that remain politically dependent, notably the French territories (New Caledonia, French Polynesia and Wallis and Futuna), and least adequate in the larger states of Melanesia, where there are proportionately fewer health workers and smaller budgets.

Other than the much larger PNG, Fiji is the largest state in the region, with about 825,000 people; the Cook Islands and Palau have fewer than twenty thousand and Niue merely fifteen hundred. Tonga and Samoa have more or less static populations, because of high rates of emigration, while Vanuatu, with almost no emigration, experiences steady population growth. The population of both Niue and the Cook Islands has fallen in recent years because of migration to New Zealand, with which they are in free association. All the island states central to the present study have experienced low or even negative rates of economic growth, most are highly dependent on agriculture, but exports are limited (and declining in the case of sugar from Fiji), and on fisheries, overseas aid, remittance flows and the vagaries of tourism. None have a secure, sustainable economic future based on national resources.

PARADISE LOST? ISLANDS IN TRANSFORMATION

During the nineteenth century the Pacific islands became better known to distant colonial powers as the last fragments of global empires were put in place, by France, the United Kingdom and the United States. By the time that Britain somewhat reluctantly acquired the Gilbert and Ellice Islands (much later to be Kiribati and Tuvalu) the lure of the Pacific had faded and these remaining islands were very much 'Cinderellas of the Empire' (Macdonald 1982). At considerable distances from the centres of empire, the activities of the colonial powers constituted an unwieldy mixture of trading, strategic and ideological pursuits, which varied substantially from place to place according to the period and manner of contact, the responses of islanders (which varied at least as much as the strategies of colonial venturers) and the location and resources of the islands. Traders took whales in some seas, sandalwood from some islands and, much later, plantation crops from many. Indian cane cutters transformed Fiji. Guns found their way to various islands, and cloth, tinned food and alcohol to almost all of them. Most islands were limited sources of economic wealth for traders and colonial powers—too small and fragmented, far from markets and with uncertain labour supplies—hence acquisition was as often for strategic reasons as economic gain.

Blackbirding, the colloquial term for the earliest forms of labour trade, was initiated as illegal recruitment and effective slavery long after such practices had ended in Europe and Africa. Some islands became sources of international labour. Labour migration was critical for Rapanui (Easter Island) and Tokelau, where many were taken against their will and perished (Maude 1981), but less problematic in the Gilbert Islands (Kiribati), where labour migration may have spared islanders becoming some of 'the first Malthusians' (Munro and Bedford 1980). From 1847 to 1872 a more extended labour trade took Melanesians to work on Queensland sugar cane plantations. Most went from the Loyalty Islands (New Caledonia), the New Hebrides (now Vanuatu) and the Solomon Islands. Eventually the British government passed the Pacific Islanders Protection Act in 1872 and blackbirding ended. After subsequent legal recruitment a small descendant population of South Sea Islanders (Kanakas) remained in Australia. In the twentieth century various forms of labour migration have involved the Pacific islands, from i-Kiribati working in the Nauru phosphate mines to Filipinos in Micronesian services, but none have involved the violence, deception and mortality rates that marked nineteenth-century blackbirding. In a sense the South Sea Islanders represent the first phase of a Pacific island diaspora.

In much of Polynesia limited domestic economic opportunities resulted in more continuous external migration. On Niue, as early as the mid-nineteenth century, the labour trade was said to have produced an 'island of women', with twice as many women there as men, after a 'mania among the young men for emigration to Samoa', and even South America (Connell 1983: 11–12). From the mid-1840s in the Cook Islands, despite attempts by the chiefs of most islands to prevent emigration, large numbers of young men left for Tahiti or the 'guano' islands on temporary labour contracts or 'sought adventure' in Sydney, Honolulu or California

(Hayes 1983). In the 1920s migration was seen as excessive by the colonial administration that recorded its disquiet for Niue in a manner that resonates in contemporary times:

> It is clear that migration and not excessive mortality is the real danger in Niue . . . The majority of the natives who are now away are now permanently domiciled in the islands in which they reside . . . some of the younger natives have even forgotten their own tongue. The prospect of seeing them again in Niue is therefore remote . . . the younger men are clamorous to go; and though they are willing to promise to return . . . such promises for the most part would not be honoured. It is only a lack of shipping that has kept men here of late. (Quoted in Bedford et al. 1980: 16)

Similar accounts were related elsewhere as a long phase of more individual migration accompanied and followed the blackbirding era.

On some islands, like those of Tokelau, the outcome of colonial contact was devastating. Banabans were displaced by mining to Fiji, and few ever saw their home island again. By contrast, the eastern islands of Fiji, if not those in the centre, supposedly 'were spared the journey through Hell' that transformed larger colonies (Knapman 1976: 183). In the Cook Islands, even more isolated from colonial influence, models of the expanding capitalism of the world system that were true elsewhere meant little, as the islands quickly became recipients of welfare rather than arenas of exploitation (Simpson 1990). Scarce opportunities for colonial economic development much later became scarce opportunities for indigenous economic development as the same factors hampered local attempts at participation in the world economy. Commercial agriculture was hindered by world prices, access and attitudes, and key commodities, such as sugar in Fiji, were propped up by preferential trade systems. Fisheries similarly failed to achieve broad economic success and the licence fees from leasing economic zones to distant states have been a more important income source. Mining was highly localized and brought few benefits to local landowners, who often resisted mining activities. Industrial development is largely absent. Tourism has flourished locally, being the sole economic sector where there is an obvious comparative advantage for islands and island states, despite its vulnerability to economic uncertainty and political instability. Most recently Pacific states have sought financial service industries but, despite its extreme flexibility and 'spacelessness', competition with established performers has been no easier in this sector than any other.

One consequence of limited economic development has been an increased resort to overseas migration as Pacific islanders have followed Caribbean precedents. Since the 1960s migration over the course of the last four decades has resulted in islanders, especially those from Polynesia, becoming urban residents in the metropolitan cities that fringe the Pacific:

> ironic as it may seem these migrants seek in the west the very things that modern day Gauguins want to leave behind—access to material goods, jobs in the industrial sector, better education for their young, and social mobility in a society they have believed free of the traditional barriers of rank and family status that made such mobility difficult at home. (Shore 1978: xii)

Migration was a safety valve for population pressures.

A second consequence of limited economic development has been a substantial dependence on overseas aid, most obviously in those island groups that retain a dependent political relationship. The decline or stagnation of the productive sector, especially agriculture, and the growth of imports offset by aid, remittances and tourist revenues, in a situation where much employment is concentrated in the public sector, has led to the conceptualization of the smallest Pacific island states as MIRAB states, dependent on Migration, Remittances and Aid which sustain the burgeoning Bureaucracy (Bertram and Watters 1995). In such states it is argued that the thrust of conventional development strategies, with their focus on increased production, is misplaced because 'aid, philately and migrant remittances are not merely supplements to local incomes, they are the foundations of the modern economy' (Bertram 1986: 809) as it moves from subsistence towards subsidy and rent. This analysis, first propounded for Kiribati, Tuvalu, Cook Islands, Niue and Tokelau, is applicable to a greater or lesser extent in most island states. Aid dependence emphasizes vulnerability. Perhaps unsurprisingly the Pacific islands are the most heavily aid-assisted part of the world on a per capita basis. The public sector increasingly dominates formal economic activity almost everywhere, despite efforts at restructuring.

Over time Pacific islands have thus been more effectively incorporated into the global and metropolitan world in a number of ways, including trade, aid, investment and migration. Movement towards the greater self-reliance that a reduction in external ties would enable would be difficult and painful. Aspirations have become firmly directed to the acquisition of modern goods, skills and education. On Rotuma 'with the prestige given to "foreign" goods, it is doubtful, therefore, that Rotumans would want to be self-sufficient even if that were a possibility' (Plant 1977: 174). In Pohnpei (FSM) too, villagers are not interested even in the rights to subsistence, but rather desire 'continued and increased access to the goods and prestige provided by employment' (Petersen 1979: 37) albeit, in both cases, with some degree of social continuity (Connell 2007d). Islands experience problems, from natural hazards to the travails of development, that have posed challenges to indigenous peoples, colonizing powers and, more recently, aid donors. Islands appear to offer distinct identities and spaces, an apparent combination of isolation and community, in an increasingly homogeneous world. However, most recently marriage, education and new forms of media have all stressed metropolitan ties, as island states have entered a world of choices and a negotiated multivariate dependence. The advertising columns of island newspapers are sadly replete with offers of marriage from distant places and the vaunted services of migration agents. It is the new diaspora that extraordinarily rapidly has come to characterize contemporary island realms.

Island geographies too have been reconstituted. Hau'ofa (1993) has challenged and replaced the remoteness and isolation of 'islands in a far sea' to envisage a 'sea of islands'. That vision, deliberately chosen to 'rekindle the sea as home' and reverse the bleakness and mendicancy implicit in the 'basket cases' of MIRAB societies, perceived the sea as link rather than barrier and contemporary migration to the metropolitan fringes of Oceania as a direct successor to the trading and settlement journeys of the distant past. Hau'ofa thus built on the great founding stories of the Pacific where heroic voyages discovered and settled new lands. Others saw this as romanticizing the past, and denying the 'safety valve' and exploitative nature and skill loss of some migration streams (Connell 2003a; D'Arcy 2006). Even so, amidst extraordinary levels of long-distance travel, and avid islander participation in Internet ties with 'home', in most island states the isolation of remote islands is as challenging as it has ever been (Morton 1999; Ward 1989), as is the enthusiasm for migration.

Prospects for contemporary economic growth are limited, especially in Polynesia and Micronesia, where no island state has a population of more than 250,000. Five island states in the Pacific (Kiribati, Samoa, Solomon Islands, Tuvalu and Vanuatu) are officially classified as least developed countries. Both the Solomon Islands and Nauru have been described as failed states (Connell 2006b; 2006c). Although the Pacific does not suffer from the absolute depths of poverty experienced in some parts of the developing world, it has significant and growing social and economic problems (Abbott 2007; Abbott and Pollard 2004). Growing populations have intensified pressure on lands and seas. Economic growth has been disappointing since independence, usually about thirty years ago, and economic stagnation has resulted in a series of imposed attempts at restructuring, urged by such institutions as the World Bank and the ADB, and directed towards smaller government and privatisation.

Globalization has posed acute economic problems for small, remote and fragmented island states with limited natural resources, human capital and domestic markets. Pacific island states have struggled to diversify and provide employment for large numbers of poorly educated school-leavers. Formal sector jobs are being created more slowly than school-leavers are emerging. The consequence is rising unemployment, a growing informal sector and visible signs of poverty, especially within urban areas. In larger cities like Suva, settlements house almost half the population: a result of rural–urban migration precipitated by the demand for services (especially education), the expiry of land leases and the breakdown of extended families. In some states urbanization and low incomes have resulted in a downward spiral—an urban 'poverty trap' from which there appears little hope of improvement and, for some urban residents, a sense of biding time, waiting for unforeseen and uncertain opportunities and sometimes securing multiple jobs, maintaining strict budgets and abandoning some 'traditional' obligations, simply to get by. Many urban residents survive rather than prosper in the city, threatened by new repressions of the poor and marginalized, in diverse anti-urban policies (Connell and Lea 2002; Connell 2003c). A parallel downward spiral may also exist in rural areas where young people choose not to enter the agricultural sector but, despite high urban unemployment, move in search of urban jobs (which their limited education often denies them), resulting in a large proportion of uncultivated land, low productivity and loss of traditional knowledge and techniques. Archipelagic populations have become increasingly concentrated on more central urbanized islands, accentuating problems of service delivery in remote areas, in turn accounting for further movement away from isolated areas and the slow depopulation of smaller, remote islands. Both urban and rural 'safety nets', where extended families supported those who experienced problems, are breaking down. Absolute poverty is increasing, but a poverty of opportunity, and even a poverty of dignity, are more critical.

Differences in economic development and welfare between island states and those of the metropolitan fringe are perceived to be increasing, hence the contemporary phase of migration from the island states to the Pacific periphery. In the past decade some of the difficulties attached to social and economic development have been reflected in political crises, particularly within the Melanesian states, and external observers have perceived an 'arc of crisis' or 'arc of instability' loosely extending from Timor and West Papua eastwards to Fiji, itself sometimes described as being absorbed in a 'coup culture'. Others have perceived 'failed states' and 'weak states' where, for example, central government holds little sway and has minimal administrative capacity in distant areas of the nation, or even at the centre, resulting in external intervention in various forms, whether as aid delivery, the restructuring of national economies or regional police and military intervention, as in the Solomon Islands (Connell 2006c). Yet there is enormous diversity within the island states, whether of culture, population size, location or development potential. The following sections provide some background to the economic and migration situation in the states where the present project was primarily conducted.

THE PACIFIC ISLAND STATES

The Heart of Polynesia: The Cook Islands and Niue

With the sole exception of American Samoa, all the Polynesian states have either declining or more or less static populations because of migration. American Samoa has become a stepping-stone for many, especially from Samoa, en route to the United States and the majority of American Samoans live there (Ahlburg and Levin 1990). The tiny French territory of Wallis and Futuna has a growth rate of 0.7 percent, only because of substantial French aid to the two islands, both of which experience migration to the much larger territory of New Caledonia. Much smaller Tokelau is equally dependent on migration, remittances and aid and has three times rejected the opportunity for greater independence from New Zealand (Connell 2009). In the Cook Islands, Niue and Tokelau populations are all falling, while Samoa and Tonga are growing at 0.1 percent and 0.4 percent respectively. Tuvalu, scattered over nine coral atolls, has experienced a declining population in recent years as migration has shifted from a temporary phenomenon (like neighbouring Kiribati, to the phosphate island of Nauru and as crew on overseas shipping lines) to a more permanent migration to New Zealand, and a greater dependence on remittances (Boland and Dollery 2007), resembling that of other independent Polynesian states. In each case economic growth is weak or non-existent and migration has long dominated demographic change.

Table 2.1 Pacific Populations

	Population	*Population density (persons per sq km)*	*Population growth rate*	*Urban population (%)*	*Total fertility rate*	*IMR*	*Life expectancy at birth*	*GDP per capita US$*
Cook Islands	14,000	80	-0.5	42	2.9	15	72.3	11,000
FSM	111,000	158	0.5	22	4.0	38	67.7	2,200
Fiji	832,000	46	0.5	46	2.6	19	65.7	8,380
Kiribati	95,000	118	1.9	44	3.5	52	61.5	790
Marshall Islands	53,000	290	1.0	68	4.4	35	65.5	1,820
Nauru	9.900	473	2.3	100	4.0	42	55.4	..
Niue	1,450	6	-2.5	36	2.6	8	71.5	8,000
Palau	20,000	41	0.6	64	1.9	31	69.0	5,700
PNG	6,333,000	14	2.2	14	4.6	64	54.3	850
Samoa	179,000	61	0.1	24	4.6	19	72.8	1,445
Solomon Islands	504,000	18	2.7	17	4.8	66	61.1	500
Tonga	102,000	157	0.4	31	4.2	19	70.2	1,780
Tuvalu	9,700	373	0.3	47	3.7	35	65.3	2,100
Vanuatu	227,000	19	2.6	22	4.4	67	67.3	1,330
Australia	20,500,000	3	1.1	87	1.8	5	80.6	15,240

Source: Based on Secretariat of the Pacific Community 2007.

The Cook Islands and Niue are two of the smallest island states in the Pacific. Neither has achieved full independence and their residents are New Zealand citizens. The majority of ethnic Niueans and Cook Islanders live overseas. The population of the Cook Islands is about fourteen thousand (but there are about fifty-eight thousand people of Cook Islands ancestry in New Zealand, alongside twenty-two thousand people of Niuean descent). The Niue population peaked at over five thousand in the mid-1960s but has slipped below fifteen hundred people, most supported through public service employment (Connell 2007a; 2008b). Limited land resources, few natural resources, isolation and fragmentation (in the Cook Islands), weak infrastructures and governance all pose problems for administration and development. The Cook Islands has an economy dependent on agriculture and tourism but Niue has no real commercial economy. Conventional development strategies through export production or even tourism have been argued to be no more than a 'prescriptive unreality' (Cohn 2003; Connell 2007b). Migration is a greater influence on social, economic and political life than in all other Pacific island states.

Two notable periods of mass international migration have affected the Cook Islands. The first was in 1978 after the airport opened in Rarotonga, making international travel easier and more affordable. The second was in 1996 when the state faced a recession and eighteen hundred public servants were made redundant. Many health workers went overseas; nurses left for Australia and New Zealand and maintenance of facilities declined. More than a hundred migrant Fijians have joined the tourist industry in recent years, but some sectors continue to experience labour shortages. High rates of emigration and immigration have posed questions about economic development, service provision and national identity and are widely seen as one of the biggest problems facing the country. As one public servant phrased it: 'migration outward and inward is the most serious problem facing the country [and] our politicians don't have a clue what to do about it' (quoted in Dusevic 2001). One Member of Parliament has said:

> Migration is the best and worst thing about the Cook Islands. Yes, there is a brain drain. But there is also the release of a safety valve. We couldn't support the number of Cook Islanders who now live overseas, and they pump a lot of money back into the country to support parents and children. (Quoted in Dusevic 2001)

Migration is substantial for both states because of the complete freedom to migrate between the Cook Islands, New Zealand and Australia.

Greater Polynesia: Samoa and Tonga

Both the larger Polynesian states—Tonga and Samoa—share many characteristics: fragmented geographies, long-established migration streams, a constant search for new opportunities and largely stable populations and economies. Samoa (formerly Western Samoa) has a population of about 170,000, two thirds of whom are on the island of Upolu, which contains the only town, Apia, and the national hospital. Uneven development is increasing as more economic activity is concentrated around Apia. Samoa is a least developed state, with a small open economy, dependent on a narrow resource base—centred on agriculture and fishing, both of which are currently declining—and on aid and remittances. About 20 percent of the population live below the national poverty line (KVA Consult 2007). The last two sources of income are much the most important in the country, emphasizing the important role of migration for the nation's economy, where as many ethnic Samoans live overseas as in Samoa.

Tonga has a population of just over one hundred thousand and, like Samoa, somewhat more ethnic Tongans live overseas: in New Zealand, the United States and Australia. Similarly, as in Samoa, the population has not grown for twenty years, migration balances natural increase, the economy has grown slowly, but both agriculture and fisheries have stagnated. The main market for Tonga's agricultural exports is overseas Tongans (Utoikamanu 2007). Imports are substantially greater in value than exports, with the difference in value being made up from remittances (which constitute at least a third of GDP) and aid. The significance of remittances indicates the key role of international migration for Tonga, and demand for migration has increased after the civil unrest of late 2006 when a significant part of the business district was burned down.

Micronesia

The British Sphere: Kiribati

Both Kiribati and Nauru have been more influenced by British colonialism than northern parts of Micronesia that came under the American sphere. Nauru is an isolated, uplifted atoll that until the start of the century had an economy entirely dependent on phosphate mining. Mismanagement and corruption turned Nauru into a failed state (Connell 2006b), and the absence of development opportunities has left the island with a bleak future, that even migration is unlikely to resolve. Kiribati is made up of thirty-three islands, almost all coral atolls, has very limited natural resources, is exceptionally fragmented, is one of the poorest states in the region and a least developed economy. Despite attempts at decentralization to the remote Line Islands, more than a third of the population lives on the overcrowded urbanized atoll of South Tarawa. A major cost to the nation is providing infrastructure and services because the population is so widely dispersed. The formal economy of Kiribati is dominated by government activity, with a small private sector largely restricted to services. Only 21 percent of the working-age population are in paid employment, mainly in South Tarawa, while the majority of the population live a semi-subsistence lifestyle. Aid, migration and remittances are extremely important to the Kiribati economy, but the migration from Kiribati is different from that in other island states since little is permanent. Kiribati, exactly like Tuvalu, is one of very few nations that train its citizens for overseas employment. The limited number of permanent emigrants means that there are few overseas support networks on which potential migrants could rely.

An American Sphere: The Marshall Islands, Palau and the Federated States of Micronesia

Four states make up what was after the Second World War the United States administered Trust Territory of the Pacific Islands (TTPI). After the American mandate was eventually withdrawn three states chose independence, while the Northern Marianas chose to retain a close relationship with the United States like its neighbour Guam. Both Guam and the Northern Marianas have been destinations for substantial migration from other parts of the former TTPI.

About half the population of Guam trace their roots to the indigenous Chamorro population and a fifth are Filipino migrants. The main source of revenue is government expenditure largely connected with American military installations, which cover a third of the island, hence almost a quarter of the population are US military personnel and their dependents, giving the island a neocolonial character quite different from most of the Pacific. Health care in Guam has been critical in recent years with overcrowding of the hospital, nurse shortages and a lack of medicines and basic supplies (Marsh 2007). The Northern Marianas have some similar characteristics to Guam, not least a situation where health services were in crisis in 2007 with some 95 percent of nursing staff being migrants and a critical shortage of doctors (McPhetres 2008: 206). American support is crucial to the economy, which largely collapsed in the early 2000s with the end of the textile industry which had brought large numbers of Chinese and Filipino workers to the main island of Saipan. Both states have fluctuating tourist economies oriented to Asia.

The three independent Micronesian states of the Marshall Islands, Palau and the FSM have had a complex colonial history involving Spanish, German and Japanese colonization, Japanese occupation during the Second World War, followed by American administration. Each of the three areas chose to move towards independence in the 1980s and 1990s by signing a Compact of Free Association (CFA) with the United States. The CFA gave the three states very substantial aid over a fifteen-year period (subsequently renewed) alongside unrestricted migration to the United States and its dependencies. Islanders have made considerable use of this provision as domestic economies have failed to develop.

The Republic of the Marshall Islands consists of twenty-six populated coral atolls. Natural resources are extremely limited, the prospects for self-reliant development minimal and the government sector dominates the economy, which is heavily dependent on United States aid. There has been no economic growth since independence and virtually nothing is exported, in a context described by the ADB as 'a uniquely dependent psychological and economic relationship with USA' (2001: viii). The Marshall Islands has an annual population growth rate of about 1.3 percent, slowing because of emigration, but one of the most youthful populations in the world. More than two-thirds of the population lives in the urban areas of Majuro and Ebeye atolls, where population densities are the highest in the Pacific region. The original CFA, renegotiated in 2002, enabled aid delivery from, and continued migration to, the United States. As the Marshall Islands Minister of Foreign Affairs has said: 'From a Marshallese perspective one of the most important benefits of the compact is the right of citizens to enter, reside, join the military, work and go to school in the United States' (*Baltimore Sun*, 15 September 2002). In the last decade this has resulted in very substantial emigration, with new overseas communities rapidly emerging (Hess, Nero and Burton 2001). Labour has been recruited under unregulated and exploitative conditions, some to work in the United States private health system, mainly in private nursing homes, at wages and conditions unacceptable to established residents.

Though Palau has an economy that is largely dependent on United States aid, it has managed to achieve more diversification than other former TTPI states and has a tourism industry, centred around diving the rock islands, strongly oriented towards Asia. Two-thirds of its population of about twenty thousand live in the urban centre of Koror. Urban population density is nearly as high as in the Marshall Islands and plans are steadily being implemented to decentralize capital city functions to a new centre on the larger island of Babeldaob. Emigration has been longer established in Palau than in the other Micronesian states, and there are substantial communities in the United States and Guam, while immigration from the Philippines and elsewhere has also been substantial and controversial (Pierantozzi 2000).

The FSM, like Kiribati one of the largest countries in the world in area, has an economic structure similar to the Marshall Islands. Four states make up the federation, with secessionist tensions between Yap and the other states. Economic growth has been weak, and even sectors assumed to have potential, such as fisheries and tourism, have failed to develop, partly because of the high costs of isolation. The modern sector, mainly services, is concentrated on the four high islands at the centre of each state, to which there has been significant migration from the outer islands. Migration to the United States has intensified in the present century and remittances have slowly become significant, although initially flowing towards migrants (Grieco 2003; Marshall 2004) alongside CFA aid. Like both Tuvalu and the Marshall Islands the structure of migration and the economy are becoming much more like that of central Polynesia.

Melanesia: The Largest States

Melanesia was one of the last regions of the world to be discovered, contacted, explored and colonized, and to become independent, with hesitation in several places and violence in Vanuatu. The Melanesian states are characterized by low population densities, cultural and linguistic diversity, a significant rural, subsistence-based population and a poorer health status than most of the Pacific. Poverty, hardship and some degree of ethnic tension and violence occur. Both PNG and the Solomon Islands have rapidly growing populations and low life expectancies, where health issues are primarily concerned with infectious diseases, malaria and tuberculosis, with NCDs being relatively slight but HIV/AIDS having reached epidemic proportions in PNG. Both countries are relatively poorly served by health services, have introduced expatriate doctors from several countries (including Cuba and Taiwan) and still remain partially dependent on mission medical services.

Unlike Micronesia and Polynesia the much larger Melanesian states are not characterized by international migration, but by internal migration and urbanization (Connell and Lea 2002). Increasingly, however, each of the Melanesian states, but above all Fiji, the easternmost with many social characteristics that are similar to those of Polynesia (thus challenging traditional cultural divisions of the region), are becoming sources of international migrants. For Vanuatu, the Solomon Islands and PNG, this has mainly meant a handful of skilled workers, but for Fiji migration now occurs across all economic sectors, regions and ethnicities (notably including the remote island of Rotuma). Simultaneously all the Melanesian states requested migration opportunities for unskilled workers in Australia and New Zealand. Since 2007 New Zealand has allowed temporary short-term employment in agriculture from several island states, including Vanuatu. In a sense there were indications that, after a century's break, Melanesia was reverting towards a more benign 'blackbirding'. Migration opportunities had become a new mantra and a new reality for the entire Pacific region.

Fiji

After PNG, Fiji is much the largest Pacific island state, with a population of around 830,000 on a hundred populated islands, and the most complex economy, heavily dependent on sugar and tourism. Just over half the population are ethnic Fijians and over 40 percent are Indo-Fijians, the descendants of the early cane cutters, and there is a significant Polynesian population from Rotuma. The sugar industry remains in crisis, for both international and domestic reasons, principally the gradual loss of EU preferences and leasehold disputes, and many displayed cane workers have migrated into urban areas. The capital city, Suva, has a population of 180,000 and is part of the rapidly growing Suva-Nausori corridor with almost a quarter of a million people.

Tourism has become the main source of foreign exchange, and an important area of employment, but tourist numbers have scarcely grown in the present century. Tourism has been highly susceptible to coups, most recently late in 2006 when the army ousted the elected government, ushering in effective military rule. The textile industry too has experienced declining trade preferences and the closure of many factories, while recently mining has effectively ended. Fiji has consequently become much more dependent on remittances as domestic income sources dwindled and migration increased. Remittances made up 6 percent of the GDP in 2007 and the volume was much the highest in the island Pacific. The economy has struggled to survive these economic and political crises, but dwindling foreign reserves and rising unemployment mark a country where a third of the population are officially below the poverty line (Chand 2007). National challenges include re-establishing a growing economy and getting rid of a 'coup culture' (Durutalo 2007) that periodically disrupts development and encourages migration.

Vanuatu

Of all Pacific island states, Vanuatu (with the Solomon Islands) is most dependent on a subsistence economy, and with PNG has the highest proportion (over three-quarters) of the population living in rural areas. Vanuatu has a rapidly growing population of 230,000 scattered over some eighty populated islands, which makes equitable health provision difficult. Fragmentation is accentuated by over a hundred languages, a measure of the cultural diversity, and a colonial history that left a legacy of French, English and a lingua franca, Bislama. Rapid population growth has meant that the population per doctor has increased by 59 per cent in twenty years. About forty thousand residents live in the capital, Port Vila. Political instability has resulted in frequent changes in government, and therefore in policy and within the bureaucracy, making medium-term policy development difficult. Services, including a small offshore financial centre, dominate the formal economy, which is almost wholly urban.

Vanuatu only exports agricultural goods, but tourism contributes over half the GDP, placing great pressure on land resources, especially around Port Vila (Henckel 2006). Guided by the ADB, Vanuatu undertook a Comprehensive Reform Program after 1997 which sought to stabilize public service numbers and improve the delivery of services especially in rural areas. As a least developed country, Vanuatu has been heavily aid-dependent and is the only Pacific island state to have benefited from the

United States government funded Millennium Challenge Fund, because of its assumed propriety and integrity. After a century, international migration from Vanuatu began again in the second half of 2007 with more than a thousand workers taking up seasonal fruit picking in New Zealand (Hammond and Connell 2009). Fiji and Vanuatu are the foremost Melanesian countries moving closer towards the Polynesian and Micronesian 'model' where migration and remittances are central to economic development.

A Population Context?

All Pacific states are going through the demographic transition but population growth remains high in some places, including the larger Melanesian states. While the average population growth rate is around 2 percent, in Vanuatu and Solomon Islands it is around 2.6 percent,though falling. In most states growth rates are less than 1 percent, mainly because of extensive outmigration. Only in Fiji has there been significant adoption of modern family planning techniques. Outside Melanesia emigration has long been the single most important regulator of demographic change, especially as modern contraception has not been easily available; hence, migration has usually been partly a 'safety valve' for both population growth and increasingly for economic stagnation.

Life expectancies have risen over the past quarter of a century, but remain lowest in the Melanesian states, being less than fifty-five in PNG but over seventy in most Polynesian states. Infant mortality rates (IMR) are also highest in Melanesia, with Vanuatu (at 67 per thousand) the worst of the region, compared with less than fifteen for most parts of Polynesia. In PNG the IMR is actually increasing because of inadequate, and declining, provision of health services to rural areas.

In certain localized contexts population pressure on resources is perceived as a growing problem. In some coral atolls, at least in Kiribati and Tuvalu, islanders were being resettled (to the Phoenix Islands and to Fiji) in the 1940s. Further resettlement took i-Kiribati to the Line Islands and the Solomon Islands in the 1950s and 1960s, and Tokelauans to New Zealand in the 1960s. In many areas population pressure on resources has created tensions, where land is not freely available, but zealously guarded by its traditional owners. More broadly it has been suggested that there is a possible correlation between recent political tensions in the Melanesian region (Fiji, Vanuatu and the Solomon Islands) and growing population pressures, since migration from these countries is limited or non-existent in contrast to the Polynesian and Micronesian states where migration has been considerable and political stability greater (Ware 2005). However, other crucial differences and indications of tensions elsewhere (notably Tonga) suggest that the relationship between migration, population pressure on resources and political tensions is much more complex.

Health and Health Care

Health status varies considerably within the Pacific and is least adequate in the large Melanesian states, compared with better financed political dependencies (Taylor, Bampton and Lopez 2005). Variations are a function of local conditions, economic and social development, the isolation of many parts of Melanesian and Micronesian states, and the status of health care. Even greater variations exist in health services provision and financing (Table 2.2). At the core of the uneven distribution of human resources, hospital beds (and other physical resources) are significant variations in funding, in absolute terms and in the proportion of national budgets spent on health care. Again there is an exceptional range, from less than US$100 per capita in seven countries (including most of the least developed countries) to over US$500 per capita in Nauru and Palau (while dependent territories such as Guam and New Caledonia spend over US$1000). Not only are these absolute sums low but they also represent small proportions of national budgets, being less that 5 percent in Vanuatu and the Solomon Islands. In every case this compares poorly with the over US$1800 in metropolitan rim counties such as New Zealand and Australia, which represents 20 percent and 17.5 percent of overall government expenditure. The proportion of budgets devoted to wages and salaries is as high as two-thirds of the total budget in several states despite high vacancy rates, lack of equipment and shortages of basic supplies. Consequently there are relatively few doctors, and low doctor to patient ratios in the same group of states. In the few cases where more detailed information is available, only a small proportion of health budgets are allocated to primary health care (PHC), but high proportions, as in the Marshall Islands, may fund referrals and expatriate workers rather than local endeavours.

The number of people per doctor ranges from under one thousand (in the Cook Islands and Niue, and in dependent territories such as New Caledonia and Guam) to almost ten thousand in Vanuatu and PNG. Similar variations and discrepancies occur in the availability of other health workers, whether nurses, dentists or pharmacists; variations are less significant for nurses, because of their generally larger numbers, but more significant for pharmacists whose numbers are few. Smaller countries like Niue, Palau and Tuvalu have only a single pharmacist. Nonetheless as the provision of SHWs in Niue indicates, the minimal need for at least one dentist and one pharmacist (and other allied workers) results in 'reverse economies of scale' that give Niue higher ratios of SHW provision than Australia. (Isolation and mainly New Zealand aid have given the island a health care system vastly superior to that in any other comparably sized island in the region, and much better than that in settlements of similar size in developed countries, including supporting infrastructure such as an ambulance which usually moves from its parking spot for no more than inspections and maintenance and attendance at the weekly airline flight at the nearby airport.)

Table 2.2 Health Status

	HDI	Health Expenditure (US$ p.c.)	National Budget on Health (%)	Births Attended by Trained Personnel (%)	Access to Safe Water (%)	Doctors per 10,000 people	Dentists per 10,000 people	Nurses per 10,000 people	Pharma-cists per 1,000 people	Hospital Beds per 1,000 people
Cook Islands	0.82	294	9.6	..	100	15	10	33	0.1	4.0
FSM	0.57	143	8.8	..	59	5	1	20	..	3.2
Fiji	0.75	61	8.3	99	65	4	0.4	20	0.07	2.1
Kiribati	0.52	95	7.8	89	64	2	0.3	27	0.05	1.5
Marshall Islands	0.56	248	14.0	..	85	5	1	29	0.04	1.7
Nauru	0.66	798	8.8	..	100	5	1	48	..	4.3
Niue	0.77	417	13.5	100	100	23	17	75	1.0	4.6
Palau	0.86	607	16.4	..	95	12	1	56	0.06	4.5
PNG	0.52	24	8.6	42	39	1	0.3	15	..	..
Samoa	0.78	94	5.6	100	88	3	0.3	7	0.03	1.4
Solomon Islands	0.59	83	4.8	43	70	2	1	13	0.07	1.5
Tonga	0.81	49	10.5	98	94	4	2	34	0.17	2.9
Tuvalu	0.58	142	6.1	..	100	4	2	31	0.09	5.2
Vanuatu	0.66	76	3.9	87	60	1	..	14	..	1.8
Australia	*0.96*	*1960*	*17.5*	*100*	*100*	*27*	*27*	*79*	*0.7*	*3.9*

Sources: WHO 2006b, 2006c. Most data are from years between 2003 and 2005. The table uses the latest official WHO data. Other sources are different. Thus UNDP (2007) has per capita health expenditure for 2006 (US$) as Fiji 284, PNG 147, Samoa 218, Solomon Islands 114, Tonga 316, Vanuatu 123 and Australia 3,123. The Human Development Index (HDI) is a summary measure combining life expectancy, literacy rates, school enrolment ratios and GDP per capita.

For most Pacific states the situation has changed relatively little in the 1990s and 2000s. Fiji and Vanuatu, for example, both experienced a worsening of doctor to patient and nurse to patient ratios, whereas in Tonga and Samoa there had been some slight improvement. However, throughout the region, even where the numbers of doctors, nurses and other medical personnel had increased, that increase was either at the same rate as, or less than, population growth. The lack of material resources for health care may include buildings, but is particularly true of supplies, while the maintenance of expensive and complicated equipment is a common problem. This is compounded by deficiencies at middle and peripheral levels in the health workforce, especially where there is a 'tradition of moving the most competent administrators or people with quantitative/computer expertise to more "important" sectors, such as economic statistics etc' (Taylor 1990: 94). That situation has never subsequently changed, as these skills remain in high demand.

National data blur regional variations as modern health care systems have become more centralized in post-independence years (see the following). Because of their more limited numbers, doctors tend to be most concentrated in central hospitals (one reason for their migration from the periphery), whereas it is more appropriate and cost-effective for nurses to provide primary care in more remote areas. Even so, a high proportion of SHWs are employed in central hospitals in urban centres, hence coverage is quite uneven. Fewer doctors and limited financial resources increase dependence on nurses, especially in rural areas, hence the attrition and migration of nurses is particularly significant. The most effective skill mix for the region is yet to be defined though nurse practitioners play a key role in several countries, including Fiji, Samoa and Vanuatu, where they are relatively inexpensive and effective (Pak and Tukuitonga 2006: 30–32, chap. 7). That mix depends on the nature and location of health problems.

A Short History

Health was early recognised to be a significant problem throughout the region, especially where population numbers were dwindling (as in parts of Melanesia), and both colonial authorities and missions gave some priority to health care though resources were never substantial. Significantly, colonial governments also trained islanders to be health workers, and in Fiji from 1889 the Native Medical Practitioners and in Papua and New Guinea in the 1930s the *doktabois*, as elsewhere in the region, were the first groups of Pacific islanders to be trained as skilled workers. In 1908 the first small group of women graduated from the Colonial Hospital in Suva as the colony's first Native Obstetric Nurses (NONs), and in 1917 the first four nurses graduated in Samoa (Barclay et al. 1998). In 1929 several Pacific colonial governments collaborated to fund a Central Medical School in Suva that trained forty students at a time (Lambert 1941: 122), while young men from Papua and later New Guinea were sent overseas on a short course at Sydney University. These early skilled workers remained firmly at the base of the hierarchy, their numbers were too few to have a significant impact on health status and the advice and assistance of most such 'modern' individuals were ignored by islanders who preferred to consult traditional practitioners.

The ideological modernity of colonial medicine only began to become significant after the Second World War when modern education was extended, urbanization and new forms of employment took islanders away from villages, but, above all, as colonial regimes ploughed more resources into developing effective and ubiquitous health care. Modern hospitals emerged in colonial capitals and islanders had new access to skilled employment in health care. Nonetheless, in fragmented island groups, far distant from most colonial powers, the resources deployed in developing health care systems and training local people were too little and very late. PNG, with more than two million people, only received its first major hospital in 1957, nurse training was entirely a mission activity until 1953 and the first proposals to even integrate mission and government health services were not made until 1972, just three years before independence. By the end of the 1960s the 'golden age' of medicine had reached the region with massive and optimistic campaigns being launched against major tropical diseases such as malaria and yellow fever and widespread assumptions that total victory was possible. Penicillin alone worked wonders. Yet without sustained investment in human resources, long-term improvements were limited.

What was then called manpower planning was in its infancy until the 1970s, the main era of decolonization. By 1970 there had been just four manpower surveys in the whole region and each of them bemoaned the lack of data and, notably in the case of Western Samoa, pointed to 'serious shortages in high-level manpower', and recognised that very limited localization had occurred (Gee 1970). Islanders often had inadequate secondary education for placement in training programmes, and it was rare to promote islanders to supervisory positions. Until 1960 no women entering nursing had more than primary school education.

Nurses were still in short supply, and resignation rates were also high, mainly as female nurses left to get married, rarely to return. Only in PNG and some parts of Micronesia were men more than a tiny proportion of nurses. By the 1970s recruits to nursing generally had secondary education (when it too became available), as countries sought to localize the bulk of nursing. Progress was slow, especially in Melanesia and Micronesia, because of education and funding constraints, complicated by nursing being derided as 'woman power', though this was one option (with one other being teaching) open to women who sought employment in contexts where other job choices might have been ruled out by parents or husbands (Manning 1970; Barclay et al. 1998). Doctors were in even shorter supply as in most colonies few achieved the educational standard required to enter medical school; in the New Hebrides (Vanuatu) in 1973 'the New Hebrides record at FScM [Fiji School of Medicine] has been one of virtually complete failure. At present there is some despair at finding candidates able to meet the FScM's entry requirement and willing to take up medicine as a career' (Bartsch 1973: 89). By the time that most countries achieved independence there was a more effective and more localized health workforce, but numbers were few. Nursing numbers were better than those of doctors because almost all countries had a nursing school, though drop-out rates were high (especially amongst those who had gone overseas for specialized training), while 'the ancillary medical staff position with regard to health service personnel other than medical and nursing is uniformly a disaster area' since the high schools produced few science-oriented graduates and the few that were produced were able to go on to 'higher positions such as doctors and nurses' rather than move into areas 'which carry no charisma of respectability' (Davidson 1980: 82). Moreover, there were only a handful of high schools—the Solomon Islands had just one—and almost a complete absence of people in mid-level supervisory and management roles. The structural weaknesses of health systems within Pacific states, already evident at independence, have resurfaced in recent years as populations and demand for improved health care provision have grown. The reductions in spending on health care systems in the Pacific, that became evident from the 1980s, have had a damaging result in sustaining a skilled health labour force and meeting national needs.

Countries are at various stages of the epidemiological transition, from a situation where the causes of morbidity and mortality are dominated by infection, acute respiratory disease and undernutrition to one where NCDs, or 'lifestyle diseases', especially cardiovascular disease, diabetes and cancer, and external causes (such as accidents), alongside URT, skin infections and gastro-intestinal problems, are the principal causes of ill-health (Lewis and Rapaport 1995). Such changes are a function of greater sedentarism and new patterns of nutrition (oriented to imported, processed foods, such as mutton flaps and noodles), often resulting in inadequate diets (Coyne 2000; Evans et al. 2002; Thaman 2003; Gewertz and Errington 2007), alcohol consumption and smoking (Kuschel, Takiika and Kiu 2005; Seniloti 2005). Substance abuse is emerging as a problem. NCDs account for up to 70 percent of all deaths in the Pacific (Ken 2007). In several parts of Polynesia and Micronesia especially there are very high suicide rates, with the Pacific, and particularly the Marshall Islands, having some of the highest rates of youth suicide in the world (Rubinstein 1992; Booth 1999; ADB 2006: 118; Jenkins and McSwain 2005). At least in Samoa this high rate has been associated with migration, in terms of both absent or declining migration opportunities frustrating local youth (Macpherson and Macpherson 1987) and the absence of parents and relatives through migration, which has resulted in customary and familial structures for socialization and dispute resolution being missing or ineffective (Hezel 1989). The first five countries listed as the world's most obese nations are all in the Pacific: Nauru, FSM, Cook Islands, Tonga and Niue, while Samoa, Palau and Kiribati are also in the top ten (Pareti 2007). In recent years there has been some re-emergence of infectious diseases, notably tuberculosis and yaws (in Melanesia) and a rise in both malaria and dengue, while the Pacific has the highest incidence of rheumatic heart disease in the world. The recent rapid growth of HIV/AIDS has reached epidemic proportions in PNG, but is also significant in Fiji and Kiribati and slowly growing elsewhere. In Kiribati, and perhaps elsewhere, the recent rise of HIV/AIDS, though still at a low prevalence rate, has also been related to greater migration, especially of seamen. PNG, Solomon Islands and Vanuatu stand at one end of the spectrum, where infectious diseases are dominant, with the Polynesian states (and to a lesser extent Micronesia) at the other, though most states share a 'double burden' of NCDs and infectious diseases. In several Polynesian states, notably Tonga (and American Samoa), the incidence of NCDs surpasses that in developed countries, while Nauru achieved the highest incidence of diabetes in the world.

Longer life expectancies, aging and growing populations, the rise of NCDs and the migration of people in working-age groups have placed increased stress on all health care systems. Almost all old people are cared for at home but, where migration has been considerable, old people have become an increasing burden as the dependency ratio increases, as it has in Niue (Barker 1994). The new hospital, completed in 2006, has dedicated a wing to the immobile old—one of the few such geriatric wings in the Pacific. The availability of SHWs, and also family, are crucial to the effectiveness of health systems.

Private Sectors

In most island states public sectors dominate and the private health sector has until recently been conspicuous by its absence. It is now growing. Small urban populations, lack of means to pay, limited privatisation of health insurance and competition from the public sector (where most services have been virtually free) meant that few private practitioners could be supported in the island states until recently. The private sector, however, extends beyond what seem the formal confines of health care since several large organizations, including the Fiji Sugar Corporation and large hotel resorts, have attracted nurses at higher wage levels than in the health system itself. Some large corporations, such as mining companies in PNG, have brought in their own private medical care systems and sometimes extended these to nearby local populations, but the emergence of a small private sector largely followed frustrations with the public sector on the part of a small local elite. The rise of a well-funded private sector, epitomized by the contrast between the gleaming Suva Private and the adjacent, dowdy Colonial

War Memorial (CWM) hospitals in Suva has resulted in the migration of SHWs into that sector, weakening the public sector.

Fiji is the only country in the region with a significant private sector (partly reflecting the number of regional organizations and expatriates based in Suva). At the end of the 1990s about 20 percent of all doctors were in private practice, along with a smaller proportion of nurses. This shift to the private sector was then seen as a critical problem for addressing national human resource needs (ADB 2000a: 219). When Suva Private first started in 2001, significant movement of SHWs into the hospital actually slowed post-coup losses from Fiji. Many SHWs, returning from training or employment overseas, have sought to shift into the private sector, where wages and working conditions are superior. Most other states have a very small private sector, with no great impact on the public sector. The Cook Islands moved towards a private hospital in 2007, intending to complement new five-star hotels and perhaps also a third of working Cook Islanders with medical insurance, though it was claimed that no islanders needing serious attention would be turned away (*Radio New Zealand International*, 12 December 2006). In Tonga and Samoa, with its twenty-one-bed MedCen hospital, small private sectors meet the needs of some expatriates and those who are willing to pay in order to avoid hospital queues. At the end of 2000 the Tongan private sector consisted of two doctors, a dentist and a pharmacist, though several public sector doctors and dentists also practiced privately (ADB 2002a: 88). Most private health care providers are government employees who run part-time clinics, many out of their own homes.

Crises in public sectors have resulted in boosts to the private sector, as doctors and nurses cross over to the private sector and patients lose faith in the public sector. In 1996 when economic reforms and restructuring resulted in various problems in the Cook Islands public sector, including deferred health facility and equipment maintenance and poor service delivery, as many people as could afford it took out private health insurance. By contrast, the Medcen hospital proved invaluable in 2005 during the Samoan doctors strike (Chapter 5), and the private sector has gradually grown. Though the private sector remains small, it has resulted in a unidirectional movement of workers from the public sector into a sector that supports a very small proportion of the local population, dominated by expatriates, and provides a model where health care is accessible to the relatively affluent.

Specialization and Referral

Small populations and scarce resources mean that specialization is not cost-effective in clinical, administrative and public health areas. In some states there is no clinical specialization at all, and in the larger countries there is some specialization into medicine, surgery and paediatrics at the national level. Tuvalu and Niue have no specialist surgeon or anæsthetist, so complex surgical cases must be referred to Fiji and New Zealand respectively. Many Directors of Health, or even Ministers, as in Tonga, may divide their time between bureaucratic management, the practice of general medicine and the performance of specialized surgical procedures. No island states have trained epidemiologists or health economists.

Self-sufficiency in medical and health resources is impossible, even with reasonably high standards of living. 'Training highly specialized clinical, administrative and public health personnel is not only an inappropriate use of resources in the less-developed island countries with small populations, it is inappropriate no matter what the level of development' (Taylor 1990: 90). This can be a disincentive for those who have, or aspire to have, particular specializations to remain in the health care system in island states (Chapter 6). Conversely, where there are very few individuals with particular expertise, whether medical or administrative, their loss to the health system because of emigration (or any other reason) is a greater loss to small island health care systems than within larger states.

One implication of limited specialization is relatively frequent international referral and evacuation. For the former American territories it has become 'big business'. In the Marshall Islands and Palau, high expectations assume that people will routinely be evacuated for diagnosis and treatment. During the early 1980s the Marshall Islands spent about half its health budget on off-island referrals, mainly to Hawaii, and about a third in the 1990s; the proportion in American Samoa was about one-third. Off-island referrals from the Marshall Islands cost US$3.7 million in 2000, approximately US$20,000 for each case (Marshall Islands 2001b), while FSM was spending more on referrals in the 1990s than on all public health programmes combined (Taylor 1990: 99; Tokuda, Cernada and Kurahara 2001). Little has changed since then despite attempts to reduce the referral rate. Referrals remain expensive, benefiting relatively well-off urban residents. In Tonga, for at least a period in the 2000s, budget provision existed for transfers and referrals overseas, but only for public servants and members of parliament. In Kiribati 'generally only expatriates and politicians are evacuated for medical treatment' (McMurray 2004: 98). Politicians similarly dominated referrals in the Marshall Islands, which were thus subject to political interference, while simultaneously emphasizing the difficulties of achieving or retaining an adequate supply of health practitioners and facilities in small island states.

In the Marshall Islands (and elsewhere) this system is often inequitable in focusing on the perceived needs of those on the two central, urbanized islands rather than those in the outer islands. As one doctor said: 'the reason we send people to Honolulu is because this hospital isn't good. But the reason we don't have a good hospital is because we send people to Honolulu. . . . we are not clear about what level of care we need in this country'. Between 2001 and 2004 the number and cost of referrals fell significantly as local diagnostic capacity improved, politically inspired referrals were reduced and more patients were sent to low-cost health providers in the Philippines rather than Hawaii (ADB 2006: 113). Fiji, with little finance for referrals, has resorted to sending some patients to India for cardiac, orthopaedic and cancer treatments because it is cheaper than Australia or New Zealand; in mid-2005 at least fifty patients were awaiting surgery in India (*Radio Fiji News*, 23 May 2005; *Fiji Times*, 21 July 2007).

As long as high levels of referrals continue, island health systems are likely to be regarded as inferior by many of the local population. Correspondingly, as long as there is a shortage of SHWs, referrals are more likely to occur (at some cost) for preventable conditions (Chapter 6). This problem has been effectively summarized by the World Bank for Samoa:

> The problem of thin labor markets and the nature of the chronic and persistent supply–demand imbalances for specific skills need to be explicitly recognized and the problems addressed directly in planning for the health sector where many high level skills in small numbers are required to support health service delivery efforts. (1994: 324)

Solutions to this problem, equally true of other public sectors in small states, have not been easy to find, though reduction in the number and cost of referrals would enable the health care system to focus more strongly on primary and preventative health care, 'which generally yield the greatest health return' (World Bank 1994: 120). This is not imminent.

External Aid Programmes

All island states benefit from overseas aid targeted at health, but also from direct assistance from visiting health teams, from charitable foundations or faith-based organizations in specialized areas, such as ophthalmology and various forms of surgery. Tonga, for example, is regularly visited by specialist teams from developed countries in such areas as eye surgery, plastic surgery, corrective orthopaedic surgery and rheumatic heart disease. The Marshall Islands too has benefited from the intermittent visits of similar specialized teams, as in February 2002, when it hosted a ten-day visit from a five-person Missionary Ventures orthopaedic team that divided its time between orthopaedic surgery and mission work. Four months later a Nepalese doctor conducted an eye and ear surgery in the outer islands in the absence of an ophthalmologist in the Marshall Islands (*Marianas Variety*, 28 July 2002). Hawaiian Rotary Clubs have regularly sent dental missions. Israeli ophthalmologists have worked in Palau (and Israel has also provided scholarships for Solomon Islands doctors). Such intermittent visits complement Pacific states' lack of specialization, limited high-level skills and scarce human and physical resources.

The extent of external support is considerable. The Sydney-based Orthopaedic Outreach works in several Pacific states including PNG, Fiji and Tonga, and like other voluntary organizations, undertakes procedures, donates equipment and supplies and provides training both in situ and for short-term placements in Australia (www.orthoreach.org.au). The Beeve Foundation of California has had a long-term goal of improving the lives and sight of Fijians, and by early 2008 had conducted their eighteenth annual mission to Fiji. With a team of around twenty medical volunteers from Australia, New Zealand and the United States they then claimed to have helped over 3 percent of Fiji's population (having, amongst other things, dispensed over eighteen thousand spectacles and undertaken a thousand cataract operations). In 2008 one of their volunteers was an Indo-Fijian doctor, Dr. Anis Yusuf, based at the Prince of Wales hospital in Sydney, who had migrated in 1975:

> I missed home very much especially in my first years overseas but then got used to it. Fiji is still my home and where my heart is and that is why I keep coming back home very year with the Beeve Foundation to help the people back home. (*Fiji Times*, 31 January 2008)

The New Zealand–based Friends of Fiji Heart Foundation has sent medical teams and supplies to Fiji since 2006. The Foundation is funded by Indo-Fijians in New Zealand, both medical personnel and businessmen, with the objective of 'assisting the poorer sections of the community in Fiji . . . to give back to the country where we all come from' (*Fiji's Business Magazine*, September 2006). Nazmeen Reddy, who had migrated to Australia in 1990, returned annually with the Australian Open Heart Surgical Team from the Sydney Adventist Hospital:

> I have never regretted making that decision to join the team and come back every year to help the local people. Although at times I have other plans of how to spend my leave, my heart always yearns to come back home and help the locals because this is where I was born, raised, educated and worked for many years before migration.

One of her main intentions was to develop the confidence and skills of local physiotherapists, following her own advanced training in Australia (*Fiji Times*, 29 June 2006). The same team had upgraded the skills of local doctors to assist in such operations.

Such services give Pacific islanders direct access to some specialized services—though only intermittently and rarely comprehensively—and reduce some of the need for particular local specializations. However, the absence of such specializations means that some services are denied. While the Australian Open Heart team was able to operate on forty-five children, sixteen were too sick to be operated on and 'will die unnecessarily. . . of the 82 children seen by the team 61 cases could have been arrested in the early stages if an open-heart surgeon and equipment were available. But there is no specialized surgeon in Fiji and that is why these children cannot undergo such surgery as it is very expensive to send them overseas' (*Fiji Times*, 19 June 2006). Travelling overseas for such an operation costs around NZ$45,000 (US$335,000). Outside Fiji such specialist services as ophthalmology are absent. After a visit from the Australian Fred Hollows Foundation Team (that treated four hundred people on the island of Ovalau alone) some six thousand cases in Fiji still awaited surgery, and it was expected that this number would grow by about eight hundred new cases a year without more national eye doctors and nurses being trained (*Fiji Times*, 7 December 2007). Though there is a high incidence of rheumatic heart disease, open-heart surgery is locally unavailable. The leader of a visiting New Zealand team, taking on fifteen patients in Samoa in 2008, noted that providing local training in such complex procedures was in itself challenging, while 'they don't stay there if we train them; they are taken up by Australia and New Zealand' (*ABC Radio*, 6 April 2008).

While most assistance comes from Pacific Rim states, disasters have brought assistance from further afield. The Solomon Islands tsunami in March 2007, when more than fifty people died, brought doctors from Ecuador, Taiwan, France, Japan, New Zealand, PNG and Australia. Korean teams have visited Fiji. Local and locally based non-governmental organizations (NGOs) also play a role in health care, particularly PHC and emergency relief. In Vanuatu, Save the Children supports the Village Health Worker project that trains local health workers. Perhaps the most famous NGO in the region is Wan Smolbag in Vanuatu, which provides a wide range of health education programmes—especially directed against STDs and HIV/AIDS, and against unhealthy practices such as alcohol consumption, smoking and substance abuse—and has health and nutrition clinics. Other organizations such as the Red Cross are engaged in emergency relief.

Governments provide some part of direct overseas medical assistance but sometimes with political undertones. The United States Pacific Partnership team provides medical, dental and also engineering assistance in various countries, including PNG, Vanuatu, Kiribati, Nauru, Solomon Islands and Marshall Islands. Services are delivered from an amphibious United States navy vessel, whose mission 'shows the support and dedication that we have for the health and stability of the regions during the four-month mission' (*Pacific Daily News*, 8 August 2007). Israel has been particularly active in the Solomon Islands and also Nauru. Taiwan has been extremely visible in health care delivery in a region where several countries alternate between political support for Taiwan (the Republic of China) and the People's Republic of China. Taiwan's International Cooperation and Development

Fund Medical Mission has sent equipment, supplies and teams of doctors to Palau, the latter described by the Taiwan ambassador as 'all volunteers who dedicate their time to provide service and care to our allies' (*Marianas Variety*, 6 June 2007), to the Marshall Islands, Fiji and the Solomon Islands, where in 2005 it also provided US$10 million for redevelopment of the National Referral Hospital in Honiara, and training programmes for both doctors and nurses in Taiwan. Cuba's expanding role is scarcely without political connotations (Chapter 6). While cultural differences may occasionally be problematic and Chinese technology is not always compatible with existing facilities, high levels of medical assistance have boosted local health and to some extent the health systems themselves.

Primary Health Care

Primary (or preventative) health care has long been widely advocated, in terms of a more equitable distribution of more appropriate resources and a greater focus on environmental health, but expectations held out in the wake of independence (Newell 1983) have only intermittently been achieved (Tenn et al. 1994). More recently the more specific notion of 'Healthy Islands' has also been advocated, with the Fijian island of Kadavu as the prototype and community participation and ecological balance being key elements (Dever and Finau 1995; Han 1996), but little came of this initiative. New directions have been hampered by weak political commitment, a dependence on historic models (sometimes engendered by the constraints of aid delivery), including the construction and maintenance of central hospitals, and lack of vision. Indeed it has been argued that:

> Governments are building hospitals, attracting more technology, increasing medical specialization, and minimally reorienting the medical curriculums for doctors and nurses, while often neglecting the needs of rural people [whilst] Physicians and other health professionals are worried that primary health care will decrease their income, status and influence. A common claim is that the quality of service will be threatened; but this can be a subterfuge. Health professionals generally have a disproportionate ownership of and access to both wealth and power and are in the self-gratifying position of being consumers of public funds and controllers of the health market. (Pollock and Finau 1999: 291)

Attempts to shift to PHC have also been cancelled out by the transfer of resources to the more demanding NCDs. What is true of Tonga is more generally true:

> The increase in non-communicable diseases (NCDs) has now reached epidemic proportions. In addition to human suffering, NCDs can have a negative impact on family economies. The loss of income due to

> disease and the cost of treating chronic conditions can put enormous strain on families and destroy years of work to improve a family's situation. Ultimately there will be a negative impact on the country's economic development as more resources have to be used for health care and productive and experienced middle-aged people in the workforce are lost to death and chronic illness. (WHO 2006a: 345)

The 'diseases of modernity', once primarily urban, are more widespread, more demanding on scarce national and household resources, and have emphasized the focus on centralized, hospital-based curative care.

Towards Centralized Health Care

Medical systems were introduced into most Pacific colonies in the nineteenth century, with hospitals in the port towns. Rural populations were poorly served, and more often by missionary endeavour, though rural clinics became more prevalent from the 1950s, staffed by local people. The relatively late arrival of medical services in several places has meant that traditional beliefs about the causes and cures of disease are common, and two models of health care persist that are both parallel and intersecting (e.g. Hamnett and Connell 1981; McGrath 1999). Outside Melanesia, however, systems based on local knowledge have largely given way to more centralized, hierarchical, introduced health systems.

At independence most countries inherited exceptionally centralized health systems, dominated by hospital-based facilities where as much as 70 percent of health budgets could be absorbed by a single central hospital, on the assumption that patients would travel there, and many conditions were amenable to curative treatment (Davidson 1980; Taylor 2008). Challenges to that system after independence brought limited decentralization, hampered in fragmented nations and by limited budgets, whereas centralization followed the modernisation of economies, and the professionalization and bureaucratization of national health services (Schoeffel 1984), alongside the overuse of tertiary facilities, because of a preference for access to doctors as providers of outpatient care, rather than the nurses of primary care facilities, easy access to higher level facilities (especially in urban centres where alternatives may not exist), lack of a functioning referral system (hence patients become their own referral system) and the absence of higher user fees (or often any user fees) in tertiary centres that gave no incentive to use services at the lowest appropriate level.

Centralization has been partly by default, because of worsening infrastructure (particularly in Melanesia) and management problems. Economic stagnation from the 1980s onwards meant there were substantial reductions in real government spending on health (World Bank 1994). In many rural and regional areas, aid posts have closed and services, including medicines, equipment and SHWs, are absent, as in PNG

(Connell 1997). Delivery of vaccines and other stores is irregular for outer islands and a critical issue in epidemics (Rafai 2006). Over time, rural residents have come to realize that access to health care and high quality services, including SHWs, is usually least adequate in remote areas. As in the Marshall Islands, health assistants in rural aid posts and dispensaries may often be absent to obtain supplies, go for training, take leave or for social reasons (World Bank 2007: 58), hence reliable service is unpredictable. In Vanuatu the number of Village Health Workers declined by two-thirds between 1991 and 1992 with the collapse of financial support for their activities (World Bank 1994: 279). In Tonga the high proportion of the budget spent on salaries, and thus at the centre, has mean that resources for maintenance and drugs have been inadequate. Thus:

> The lack of funds for hospital maintenance can be seen in the urgent need for dental equipment and furniture at Vaiola [central] hospital and in the fact that many of the beds, mattresses and bed linen at [provincial] Vava'u Hospital are unfit for use. But the real impact of declining percentages spent on maintenance and drugs is to exacerbate the low proportionate spending on primary health care. . . . The attraction for patients of Clinics and Centres lies not in the surgical or advanced diagnostic skills of the staff but in the advantage of a local clinic being able to prescribe basic drugs, use simple diagnostic equipment, undertake home and follow-up visits and travel the local district undertaking preventive and health education programs. These are precisely the activities restricted by declining budgets for drugs, equipment, maintenance, and other vital non-salary items. The result in Tonga has been a classic case of inadequate funding for the non-hospital part of the system, low utilization of health centres and clinics because of perceived low quality of treatment, pressure and overcrowding in hospital outpatient facilities, and a failure of the primary health care system to become better oriented towards the newer lifestyle diseases. (ADB 1996: 121)

Similar urban biases towards hospitals occur elsewhere to the detriment of residents of remote areas, causing overcrowding in central hospitals and the gradual assumption that inequity is the norm.

Urban bias in health expenditure and personnel distribution is unsurprising in the Pacific where the headquarters of the health department and the main referral (or only significant) hospital are located in the capital city, which is sometimes the only significant town. This deficiency, at least in terms of the distribution of personnel, is well documented in the case of Vanuatu where the two main hospitals were relatively well supplied with staff, whereas the provincial hospitals lacked many skills (including emergency nursing skills, physiotherapy and rehabilitation skills) and the provincial health centres 'demonstrated a dramatic increase in clinical and treatment skills gaps' (Vanuatu Ministry of Health 2000). In Samoa there was a massive centralization of health care beginning in the 1970s. Between 1970 and 1978 the number of doctors in the district hospitals fell by half (from twelve to six) while the central Apia hospital gained four for a total of twenty-five, while regional health budgets changed in the same way (Hoadley 1980). Such situations are common elsewhere.

Information on the distribution of disease burdens and mortality rates within Pacific island states is largely absent; hence, it is impossible to determine where regional needs for medical care are greatest. Though 'modern' NCDs tend to be concentrated in urban areas, and some epidemics (including cholera in two Micronesian urban areas in the past two decades) are more common there because of poor environmental health (Connell 1989), higher IMRs occur in some outlying areas, emphasizing the presence of the 'inverse care law'.

Organization of health administration is necessarily hierarchical, but emphasized by sometimes authoritarian and centralized administrative structures, inherited from colonial times, producing what has been described as a 'militaristic and inflexible bureaucracy' (Taylor 1990: 105; cf. Finau 1988) that may appear, and sometimes is, autocratic to those in subordinate positions. The combination of hierarchy, authoritarianism and some degree of autocracy in health care systems where the opportunities for promotion may be few, simply because there are few higher level positions, frustrates those at lower levels in the hierarchy. Indeed, 'the criteria for promotion or demotion become largely unrelated to technical ability, qualification or organizational needs' (Finau 1988: 140), which can stimulate emigration (Chapter 5). In such hierarchical systems centralized authorities tend to monopolize planning, budgeting and human resource recruitment and allocation functions, and are reluctant to assist in capacity-building and devolution of specific functions, and the appropriate development of outlying areas.

Such bureaucratic systems are also poorly equipped to deal with the flexible specialization required in small island states, yet the small size of the bureaucracy emphasizes personal relationships. Taylor has observed of health managers that: 'In fact they live and work closely together for most of their lives. This makes many aspects of administration easier since each is familiar with the strengths and weaknesses of the other. The existing personal relationships through the health department often assist with the promotion of a sense of teamwork' (1990: 107). Yet such intimate personal and professional relationships are not always so harmonious, and tensions in the senior levels of bureaucracy are not unusual where few possibilities for change and restructuring exist. In certain circumstances there may even be a 'power struggle between the professional staff, who are directly involved in the productive process, and the management who become overly concerned with internal efficiency' (Finau 1988: 137). In such contexts the goals of achieving holistic health care are lost within personalized bureaucratic structures.

In the Provinces

The geography of the Pacific has ensured that a critical issue is rural and regional service delivery. Health care is highly uneven while, because of small size, the institutional structure is different from that in larger, less fragmented nations, so that 'reverse economies of scale' are not unusual. Particular problems relate to the delivery of health services beyond urban centres, especially in Melanesia, where funding and infrastructure are least adequate but also in very fragmented states, such as the Marshall Islands and Cook Islands, and by default where budgets are urban biased. Because of centralization people who are not too far from hospitals choose to bypass primary facilities to secure high quality facilities, as in urban Kiribati (World Bank 2007: 55). Consequently, urban hospitals tend to serve primarily urban patients; in Vanuatu some 98 percent of all hospital inpatients come from the towns where the hospitals are located, because residents of distant islands incur high costs in travelling into towns (and consequently may also see hospitals as a place of last resort and even, as in parts of PNG, a place of death). Transport in circumstances where infrastructure is particularly poor can be detrimental to health, especially with belated resort to distant facilities. Transport costs in the Marshall Islands, Fiji, Tonga and Vanuatu are a major deterrent to using urban services (World Bank 2007: 64; ADB 1996: 119–120). This unequal access emphasizes urban bias and inequity in service provision.

At its simplest, in the Cook Islands, 'physical access on the Outer Islands to the clinic services is not usually a problem except when petrol shortages restrict the ability of the staff to visit sick patients' (SAGRIC International 2000: 18). Elsewhere the lack of access to necessary goods and services runs far beyond petrol and has weakened the ability of health care systems to deliver effective services and intensified the frustrations of those professionals who work there. Generally, therefore, most SHWs in outer islands originate from those islands (Chapter 5). As a consultancy report on the Cook Islands concluded, though the nurses in outer islands themselves were well qualified,

> They need regular updates on clinical care and drug advances similar to doctors. They need regular visits (quarterly) from doctors to monitor ongoing and difficult cases. They require dependable and modern equipment to fulfil their clinical roles. Many of the Nurse Practitioners were tired and found having a break very difficult to organise due to problems getting relief staff. (SAGRIC International 2000: 29)

In such circumstances the lack of facilities was seen to reflect on the ability of the nurses to perform their duties and local communities lost confidence in the health care system, with an overall decline in morale.

Nonetheless, only two of the Cook Islands (both with populations less than five hundred) are without a resident doctor, a very different situation from that in Vanuatu or Fiji. The concept of 'outer island', formally (but relatively recently) recognised in some states such as the Marshall Islands and FSM, emphasizes acute distinctions in service provision. Significantly 'outer' islands are not very far from the centres; in most states, such as Fiji, Kiribati, Tonga and Marshall Islands, they are less distant than the horizon from the capital city. In Vanuatu even the northern half of the main island of Efate is sometimes spoken of as an 'outer island', in terms of its poor infrastructure and access to the centre.

In many Pacific island states telemedicine (telehealth) is regarded as a possible solution to some of the problems of limited finance, inadequate human resources, isolation and fragmentation, both for distance learning and diagnosis, but this is far from imminent because of the high costs of the appropriate technology (Smith 2004). In Tonga, telemedicine 'is currently but a dream' (Kupu 2000: 54; cf. Adam 2000) though in Pohnpei State (FSM) internet diagnosis has significantly reduced some health care costs, where international referrals represent 10 percent of the state's health budget and serve 1 percent of the population (Hedson 2000), and in the Cook Islands some of the southern group of islands are linked to the main island of Rarotonga for health assessments, basic management and ease of access to laboratory results.

Training

Training of health personnel in and for small states raises various problems. Most states, other than the smallest (like Niue), have nursing schools, but training medical practitioners poses greater difficulties. There are just two institutions for medical training in the Pacific: the University of Papua New Guinea and the FScM in Suva. Low secondary education standards have proved barriers to entry or completion of courses (Taylor 1990: 91). In several states, notably the Marshall Islands and Nauru, high school leavers are ill equipped even for training for specialized employment, and more than half of the skilled health workforce in some states are expatriates (WHO 2006a: 197). Many rural recruits come to urban centres for training and then marry, some never to return to rural areas, thus it has been argued that 'it may be necessary to find jobs in the health department (such as maintenance) for husbands of nurses in order that they will return to the rural setting' (Taylor 1990: 91), an indication of the significance of family factors in employment and migration and of the difficulty in maintaining adequate health care systems in rural areas. However education levels in some regional areas tend to disqualify applicants from there.

Many islanders have gained access to medical schools in Australia, New Zealand and the United States. Over a decade ago, it was possible to conclude that: 'Sophisticated medical training such as this is often inappropriate since the technology on which it is based is not available in many Pacific island countries, and graduates of these medical schools have a particularly high non-return rate' (Taylor 1990: 91). This is now less valid, because of the development of courses within the region (Oman 2007), with scholarships oriented primarily to those who live there, but some doctors continue to be trained overseas. Training of paramedical workers such as radiographers, physiotherapists and laboratory technicians also poses difficulties since relatively few such workers are needed, hence courses are either run intermittently or training is overseas. 'Some small countries may require only one or two of a certain type of personnel, but if one migrates or dies unexpectedly the workforce is decimated' (Taylor 1990: 91). The migration of such specialized personnel is usually a more acute problem for island states than the loss of doctors and nurses, simply because numbers are few and replacement is difficult.

It is unusually difficult to replace skilled migrants, because of the duration of training that is required and the limited demand for some particular skills. A report on the health workforce in Tonga observed:

> With the resignation of one physiotherapist from the Physiotherapy Unit staff earlier this year, the unit is staffed by only one qualified physiotherapist. The remaining staff member . . . has been an employee of the Ministry for the past 18 years. The unit has been without a second physiotherapist for many months—the physiotherapist who had been studying overseas did not return to Tonga on completing her training. . .. There is no likelihood of recruiting a Tongan national to fill the vacant physiotherapist post within the foreseeable future. Recruitment of a school-leaver to a newly created post of physiotherapy aide is required . . . The employment of this aide does not of course answer the need to train a second professional physiotherapist. It will be necessary to select a student to go to FScM to complete the physiotherapy diploma course there as soon as possible. (Dewdney 2000)

Similar observations were recorded for other specialized health positions, including pharmacy and radiology, and can as easily be made elsewhere. In Vanuatu the principal skills that were missing in the two main urban hospitals were non-clinical skills, including planning and management, budget control, statistical analysis and IT skills (Vanuatu Ministry of Health 2000). In Tonga not only was there no immediate prospect of gaining a recruit to go to FScM, so that the 'as soon as possible' was indefinite, but the whole procedure was utterly unpredictable. While this is less likely to be true for nurses and doctors since numbers are larger, it is even truer in smaller states. Moreover, because of the necessity for appropriate skilled training, it is more difficult to substitute for (or transfer from elsewhere in the public service) absent skills in the health workforce.

Postgraduate specialized medical training was entirely undertaken in metropolitan states until the end of the 1980s. It often required many years, was accompanied by high levels of failure and resulted in high non-return rates amongst the few who were successful (Taylor 1990: 92). A key mechanism for minimizing the excessive migration of health professionals from island states was therefore: 'As much local training in the home country, or other Pacific island countries . . . and local Master degrees for specialist qualifications is one of the answers' (ibid.). Since then new courses have been established in the region to reduce costs, ensure relevance and minimize migration and attrition.

Regional Diversity

Island states with strong political relations with metropolitan states have better funded health care systems, both in infrastructure and human resources. The health care system in the Cook Islands is extensive, given the small population of the country. This has largely depended on New Zealand aid and hence relatively higher wages and better conditions than might otherwise be expected in a country of this size and economic productivity. The major hospital for the Cook Islands is in Rarotonga, and health care needs are less well met in the northern islands. Dentists are rare outside Rarotonga, and the Ministry of Health (MOH) has hired 'flying dentists' to deal with outer island dental problems (WHO 2006a: 58). The health status of Cook Islanders is superior to that in most other island states and is comparable to that of New Zealand. Niue is similarly relatively well served, but a growing incidence of NCDs has meant a significant number of referrals to New Zealand. It has an entirely centralized health care system, based at the Niue Foou hospital, completed in 2006 and absorbing about a third of a NZ$20 million (US$15 million) New Zealand Aid (NZAID) project to restore infrastructure to the island after the previous hospital was destroyed by Cyclone Heta two years earlier. Constructing such a costly building for a state with a declining population, already much smaller than most New Zealand country towns with much poorer facilities, emphasized 'reverse economies of scale'.

Fiji has much the largest and most complex public health care system in the region, with eighteen hospitals, nearly three thousand employees and a growing private sector. Two-thirds of the health budget represents wages, salaries and related costs. A shortage of doctors first became evident in the country around 1977 when some local medical graduates resigned to run their own private medical clinics. Prior to that, graduates of the FScM were not allowed to practice in the private sector (Tuqa 1999). Ethnic tensions and military coups prompted a series of resignations and departures of SHWs, notably after the 1987 coups (Mitchell 1988) and again in 2000. The two 1987 coups, construed by many as opposition to the growing political role of the Indo-Fijian population, prompted a political, economic and social crisis and very substantial emigration, not only of Indo-Fijians. Whilst the circumstances were exceptional, one hundred doctors migrated in a period of twelve months compared with the loss of sixty-seven in the previous five years.

> This in itself has put a tremendous strain on the remaining doctors and on the health system as a whole. There has been some help in the form of doctors from China and Australia . . . but unfortunately it will take many years to recover the lost expertise and personnel. An indirect result of the loss of doctors has been the inability of doctors in Fiji to go overseas for further study. Hence we cannot expect many doctors to gain postgraduate qualifications in the next few years. Many of the doctors who have left were young people who had returned to Fiji in the last eight years because they could see some real challenges for bettering the standard of medicine here. This represents a real loss. Similarly a substantial number of nurses and other medical support staff have been lost to Fiji. In private practice, too, some doctors have migrated, leaving many people without a family doctor. (Mitchell 1988: 77)

There was not just a substantial loss of a large number of doctors and other medical workers, but those who went were some of the more competent and dedicated staff. The 1987 coups were something of a precedent for subsequent coups and new migration streams.

The health of the Kiribati population is poor in comparison with most other island states though the government provides free national health services. Because of the extremely low employment rate in the formal sector, there are no private medical practitioners. For one of the poorest states in the region, government expenditure of US$95 per capita on health is fairly high by Pacific standards. Kiribati has one major 120-bed hospital, the Tungaru Central Hospital, donated by the Japanese government, alongside twenty-four health centres, one on each inhabited island, each operated by a medical assistant. Due to the concentration of more advanced health care facilities and personnel in South Tarawa, there are 'substantial differences . . . in terms of access to qualified health personnel and level of facilities available' within Kiribati (Government of Kiribati 1999: 119). If SHWs in Kiribati wish to work elsewhere they must either leave the health profession, or migrate, not having the option of moving into the private sector or to another hospital.

Health care in the Marshall Islands is mainly provided by the government at the Majuro and Ebeye hospitals, with about eighty and thirty beds respectively, and the sixty health centres on outer islands. Health care expenditure is heavily dependent on external sources, with fully 42 percent of the funding coming from the United States (ADB 2001: 55). The proportion of the budget spent on health is one of the highest in the region, largely because of numerous referrals, and raised expectations of health care (towards American levels). There is no contemporary private involvement in health care, nor are there private pharmacies or dentists. Both communicable and NCDs are prevalent. The Marshall Islands is one of only two countries in the region (the other being FSM) where leprosy still occurs, while between 2001 and 2004 the number of diabetics hospitalized rose by 300 percent and the country also had the highest tuberculosis level in Micronesia.

Medical personnel, and the whole of the health system, are concentrated in the two main islands. No doctors or nurses have been based in any of the outer islands, few of which have populations larger than a thousand, though in 2002 a recent migrant doctor was appointed to the newly created Outer Island Dispensary System to travel between the outer islands and provide health care and also training for outer island health assistants. The Marshallese health system experiences major shortages of local staff, and continues to substantially rely on foreign health workers, with 'the two biggest hospitals largely run by expatriates, a situation that could be financially infeasible in the long run' (World Bank 1994: 133; ADB 2001). In 1994 twenty doctors and dentists were in the Marshall Islands, only two being Marshallese; the others were from the United States, the Philippines, Fiji, Sri Lanka and other Pacific countries. In 2002, a similarly high proportion of doctors and dentists were expatriates, from the same range of countries, alongside Burma and Nepal, and that dependence has not subsequently declined.

The health care system of Palau is largely centralized around an eighty-bed hospital in Koror, opened in 1992. 'In recent years health services have become concentrated in Koror. The network of rural dispensaries had been underfunded, erratically staffed and poorly managed' (United Nations 1998: 118). NCDs are the leading causes of mortality. Palau allocates some 16 percent of the national budget to health care, the highest proportion in the region, but a large proportion of this supports referrals. The MOH staff includes about twenty-two doctors, three dental officers and ninety registered and licensed nurses. Many key positions, notably doctors, are held by expatriates. As the United Nations observed:

> Palau has a critical shortage of professional nurses . . . The preferred solution is a local training program for professional nurses at Palau Community College but this is an expensive option. Until resources can be found to launch this program, the only feasible alternative is to encourage Palauans to enter foreign training programs and to offer sufficient inducements to encourage return upon their completion of training. (United Nations 1998: 118)

At that time 'wages and benefits in Palau [were] not competitive with those of the Northern Marianas [Saipan], resulting in many Palauan nurses staffing Northern Marianas facilities while Palau recruits from Fiji and Asia to maintain essential services' (ibid.). Palau has continued to recruit nurses, and a growing number and proportion of the nurses are from overseas, especially from Fiji. Palau has found it even more difficult to produce medical practitioners, a situation generally true in Micronesia.Secondary educational institutions produce few students who could qualify for appropriate courses. Few who have gone to the FScM have graduated. About fifteen Micronesians (from Palau, the FSM and the Marshall Islands) graduated from the University of Hawaii School of Medicine in the twenty year period 1970–1990, but the majority remained in the United States. Like most very small states Palau has particular difficulty with the supply of SHWs in more specialized areas:

> As is the case in virtually all Pacific nations, Palau has a serious shortage of dental personnel . . .The only option remaining is to encourage young Palauans to enter overseas dental training programs and to follow with sufficient salary and other inducements to encourage their return to Palau upon completion of training. (United Nations 1998: 118)

This has never been achieved and many skilled activities, not only in the health sector, continue to be undertaken by expatriates.

In Samoa health care is centred around the main hospital in Apia, with two small hospitals in rural Upolu, the main island, and two others on the second island, Savai'i. A small private hospital in Apia is owned and operated by two local doctors. Unusually within the Pacific the government has provided some financial support to ease pressure on the public sector (ADB 2000b). People in rural Upolu tend to travel directly to the national hospital, for what they perceive to be better health care, resulting in a decline in the use of health centres. Consequently their effectiveness has declined even further, at some cost to the relatively poor. Typhoid and dengue periodically reach epidemic levels, but NCDs, including diabetes and obesity (Hodge et al. 1994), as elsewhere in Polynesia, now represent the critical health problems, especially in Apia. Youth suicide remains a problem in Samoa (WHO 2006a). The rise of NCDs has also contributed to a parallel rise of referrals overseas, mainly to New Zealand, which by the end of the 1990s was absorbing as much as 10 percent of recurrent health expenditure (ADB 2000b; World Bank 1998), perhaps the highest figure outside Micronesia. The Department of Health has a workforce of about three hundred, and like many other health sectors is one of the largest employers in the Pacific. Most doctors and nurses are Samoans, but staff shortages are a constant problem. In 1998 as many as 30 percent of all doctors were above retirement age (ADB 2000b: 132), as were about a third of all nurses.

Tonga has a higher standard of health than most island states despite relatively low real expenditure on health care. Immunization rates are above those in many developed countries. NCDs have become the greatest problem: obesity, diabetes and cardiovascular diseases have all reached epidemic proportions, with prevalence rates above those in developed countries, partly because of very substantial consumption of imported foods (WHO 2006a: 339–340). Tonga's health system is more decentralized than in most states, but scarcely matches the national population distribution over some forty islands. Three community hospitals are in outer islands. Referrals to the central Vaiola hospital are limited, because of transportation problems. However, since about 70 percent of the country's population now live on the main island of Tongatapu, and half of these live in the capital, Nuku'alofa, the central Vaiola hospital plays a crucial role in health delivery. About 89 percent of all health expenditure takes place in the four hospitals (WHO 2006a: 344). The MOH has about four hundred established posts, but up to 25 percent of these are usually unfilled.

Vanuatu has achieved substantial improvements in health status but communicable diseases remain and life expectancy is low. Limited investment in health in real and proportional terms has resulted in a shortage of skilled workers, poor infrastructure and outdated facilities and equipment. Vanuatu has some of the highest incidences of malaria and tuberculosis in the Pacific region, and malaria is the major cause of morbidity. NCDs are becoming more common in urban areas, but only 7 percent of admissions to Vila Central Hospital are NCD related (UNDP 2005: 34). As in other Pacific states, health care is focused on curative rather than preventative health care. Health care is somewhat centralized on the two main islands of Efate and Santo, with the two major hospitals, but there are three others. In a fragmented, least developed state, decentralization of health care has been particularly difficult, and there are clear disparities between the main island of Efate and even the largest outer islands such as Santo and Tanna. The Tafea province, centred on Tanna, had one health worker per 2,360 people in 1990, about a third of the national average, and the area has been seen as 'a hard place to encourage improved health practices' (United Nations 1996: 65). As elsewhere in Melanesia, nurses and doctors do not necessarily speak the languages of the patients.

Over two hundred nurses are the core of the health system and the nucleus of staffing in the five hospitals, alongside about fifty nurse aides. Nurses are trained in Port Vila, but since a public servants strike in 1993 there has been no effective provision for in-service training for nurses, while

> Vanuatu has a long-term shortage of nurses. This is partly due to the lack of proper workforce planning for the Ministry of Health. The retirement age for public servants is the age of 55 years. However, sometimes nurses are kept until they are older because of the lack of funding to pay for their retirement benefits. (Vanuatu 2000)

Attrition of nurses has not been a problem in Vanuatu, but there has been concern over their effectiveness because of flaws in the training programme.

According to one senior health bureaucrat: 'What we have here in Vanuatu due to political and economic factors are inexperienced nurses being accelerated through a programme which lacks rigour. Also there are no senior nurses who can act as role models of PHC. The nurses often work in isolation and it is terrifying' (quoted in Kerslake 1993: 66). Budget constraints prevent adequate staffing levels, with levels in provincial hospitals averaging one nurse per thirty beds rather than a desirable level of about one to five, a situation that has led to overwork, low morale and a reduced standard of health care (ADB 2002b: 242). By 2006 there were some twenty vacancies for nurses at the main Vila Central Hospital out of a total establishment of seventy, resulting in a situation where often only one nurse and one nurse aide were on night shifts; consequently, a further 25 percent of the nurses were on sick leave or performing at less than optimal capacity because of the severe workload (Chapter 6). At health centres and dispensaries similar situations recur, hence many nurses undertake higher duties and procedures for which they are unqualified. With little supervision and few opportunities for refresher courses many nurses feel unsupported and poorly appreciated (Rotem 2007). Moreover, continued rapid population growth challenges health provision. While fourteen new dispensaries were built between 1998 and 2001, to keep up with population growth, it was not possible to fully staff them.

By contrast just fifteen doctors provide medical services in Vanuatu hospitals. At the start of the 1990s there were only five indigenous (ni-Vanuatu) doctors in the system 'and little prospect for significant localization of the workforce . . . unless there is a concerted training effort and salaries are adjusted to become competitive with those in the broader Vanuatu labor market' (World Bank 1994: 281). This never happened, and in 2002 only about ten ni-Vanuatu doctors and dentists were in the public sector with one in private practice. Hence, Vanuatu remains heavily dependent on expatriate doctors, though in 1999 nearly half the small number of practicing indigenous ni-Vanuatu doctors lived and worked outside Vanuatu: in Australia, Tonga and PNG (Hassall and Associates International 1999; ADB 2002b: 243). Some well-qualified ni-Vanuatu, including those with postgraduate qualifications, have returned to take up specific positions only to be redeployed to duties not directly related to their training. A 'significant proportion' of ni-Vanuatu doctors who have trained in PNG and elsewhere have not returned, hence the World Bank concluded: 'The bonding of students sent both for undergraduate and postgraduate training should be instituted. It may also be possible to reach agreement with neighbors (e.g. PNG and Fiji) that they will not recruit ni-Vanuatu doctors trained in these two countries, at least until they have fulfilled the bond' (1994: 281, 299). With one of the highest doctor to patient ratios in the region, this loss of skills constitutes a particular problem, and the Vanuatu health system has traditionally depended on expatriates to a greater extent than other countries in the region. Salaries have absorbed a particularly high cost of the health budget, hence 'the health sector is facing a severe crisis which will take radical action to resolve' across a range of areas (ADB 2002c: 235).Within the Pacific, Vanuatu is a critical example of the problems that follow underfunding of health care systems.

Out of Diversity

Small Pacific island states continue to confront significant health challenges ranging from continued infectious diseases and the spread of malaria, in Melanesia especially, to the rise of NCDs in Polynesia and Micronesia. Most states experience something of a double burden. Less tropical states with substantial aid levels, notably Niue and the Cook Islands, have fewer health problems and better funded health services. Almost all health care is publicly funded, and household spending is trivial, but small national economies are weak and external aid is crucial. Challenges include 'the unfinished agenda in achieving the MDGs [Millennium Development Goals], high fertility rates, continued prevalence of communicable diseases and emerging threat of HIV/AIDS, combined with a rising, and in many cases a crisis in, NCD prevalence' (World Bank 2007: vii). Urban facilities are invariably far superior to those in remote areas; centralization, urban bias and the availability of SHWs have emphasized the discrepancy. Priority areas such as PHC have failed to take off and rural and regional problems have grown, as health budgets have tended to support salaries, curative care and overseas referrals, which jointly take up around 70 percent of the recurrent health budget of Pacific island states and tend to benefit the better off leaving little for primary care and public health services (World Bank 2007: 22). Such diverse issues occur in a context where the migration of SHWs has become of much greater significance and posed new problems for poorly staffed, managed and funded health sectors. Over 15 percent of Pacific island doctors and nurses have migrated to the United States, New Zealand, Australia, the United Kingdom and neighbouring island countries in the past two decades and this trend is expected to continue. As much as anything else this creates an underlying, yet ultimately indefinite, challenge for all health care systems, where migration, in diverse forms, has become increasingly important throughout the region.

3 The Rise of Pacific Migration

In the second half of the twentieth century, migration in the Pacific went through a series of transformations, culminating in this century with migration being of almost universal importance. Until the 1950s, in Melanesia especially, migration was either typified by waves of male labourers moving to coastal plantations, remaining there for three or four years and returning to the villages and agricultural life they came from, or by a very limited movement to the small towns that were the colonial centres. Little else was possible. Melanesian towns were for colonial authorities, villagers were unwelcome and a crude apartheid even existed. In Micronesia, under Japanese rule, mobility was more frequent, as it was in Polynesia, where there was a tradition of overseas travel for young men, often as ships' crew. Micronesian and Polynesian towns were as small as those in Melanesia and were just as much places where islanders had only a tenuous connection.

In the post-war years urban segregation declined, and education and other services were extended as colonial powers took on greater responsibilities, even as colonies moved towards independence. Bureaucratic jobs, including jobs in the slowly expanding health services, became available, the first limited industrialization started and towns began to grow. They remained tiny. Nuku'alofa had reached about sixteen thousand by 1964 and Apia had grown to 21,700 in 1961. In Micronesia towns barely existed until the 1970s, when explosive growth created urban Majuro and South Tarawa. Similarly in Melanesia, both Honiara and Port Vila, the capitals of Solomon Islands and New Hebrides (Vanuatu), had less than three thousand people at the start of the 1970s, the decade of independence. Only in the immediate prelude to independence and in its wake did towns grow more quickly. In Melanesia independence coincided with the decline of plantation economies and the shift of migration streams towards the towns, in what quickly became 'over-urbanization' as towns and especially capital cities grew faster than the ability of employment, housing and health services to cope with the migrants. Growing urban permanency, high unemployment and increased expectations subsequently intensified pressure on urban services.

Internal migration was characterized by movement away from remote islands and isolated rural areas, particularly to the more central urbanized islands, such as Tongatapu in Tonga, Upolu in Samoa and Efate in Vanuatu. This emphasized problems of service delivery in remote areas, a 'vicious circle' which in turn accounted for some movement of SHWs away from isolated areas (Chapter 5). Centralization is inevitable at some scale, and the more educated have tended to migrate first. Migrants left many rural areas to take advantage of superior urban educational and employment opportunities and, more recently, out of increasing real and relative rural immiseration. While urban migration may be a lottery, within the Melanesian states especially, where international migration is absent, remittances from urban to rural areas continue to play an important role, especially for outlying islands. Even for remote parts of such large islands as Tanna, remittances from urban migrants are the single largest source of income in several villages.

Consequently migration, whether national or international, is often best seen 'as an almost inevitable decision that they [villagers] will have to make sooner or later and once this view is accepted a sort of migration momentum develops' (Walsh 1982: 7). The spreading taste for commodities has influenced work habits, and, for many in the Pacific, the largest cities and the metropolitan countries exercise a powerful allure, offer a sense of future and simply validate migration. In urban areas, especially in Melanesia and Micronesia, as in many international contexts, return migration was constantly deferred ('until children leave school', 'until enough money is saved', 'until retirement' etc.) until the point where it became implausible.

Since the 1960s in Polynesia and the 1990s in Micronesia, as urban economic opportunities have stagnated or dwindled, internal migration and urbanization have lost their allure, and have become of dwindling importance relative to international migration. Only in Kiribati and Tuvalu, where the two former British colonies have been unable to acquire obvious migration destinations, and in Melanesia does urbanization remain significant. For the rest of the Pacific urbanization has been a precursor for more significant international migration, bypassing national capitals for the cities of the metropolitan rim, and encompassing skilled and unskilled alike.

INTERNATIONAL MIGRATION

In Polynesia particularly, with its lengthy tradition of overseas migration, the small capital cities with few employment opportunities were largely bypassed by a new wave of international migration. By the 1960s the early phases of the long boom in the west had produced rapid employment growth in countries like New Zealand and Australia, and in the United Kingdom on the other side of the world, and new demands were going out for migrants, often to colonies. No longer were workers required for plantations, as in the era of blackbirding nearly a century earlier, they were now needed for the growing industrial sector. Islanders migrated as factory workers, becoming a new industrial proletariat in metropolitan cities. This new wave of unskilled workers and their families became the beachheads for others to follow.

The growing extent and significance of migration within and from the Pacific island states resulted in absolute population declines in some of the smallest states. Many moved from Niue, the Cook Islands, Tokelau, Tonga and Samoa to New Zealand (whence some went on to Australia) and to the United States. A parallel migration stream took Indo-Fijians to several metropolitan destinations, including Australia, New Zealand and Canada. In the 1990s a quite new but substantial movement of Micronesians from the small island states of Marshall Islands and the FSM to the United States and its dependencies (especially Guam and the Northern Marianas) followed the signing of the CFA (Chapter 2). Only the Melanesian states have yet to play a significant role in contemporary international migration.

For small states like Niue, American Samoa, Tokelau and the Cook Islands the majority of islanders born there now live overseas. Over two hundred thousand ethnic Samoans live overseas, more than the combined population of American Samoa and Samoa. Similarly more Tongans live overseas than live in Tonga, but for both states a significant proportion of such 'Tongans' and 'Samoans' were born overseas and some have never seen their 'home country'. Some 60,000, 23,000 and 7,000 people respectively of Cook Islands, Niuean and Tokelauan ancestry live in New Zealand, with others in Australia and elsewhere. By the early 1980s every single American and Canadian state hosted some Samoans. Significant migration from Fiji, like that from Polynesia, began in the 1970s, and unlike most other Pacific migration streams included Canada. Intermittent coups boosted emigration, especially of Indo-Fijians, which became more diverse and more wide-ranging in the 2000s. Between 1990 and 2003 some seventy-one thousand people emigrated from Fiji. Over one hundred thousand Fijians and Indo-Fijians live overseas, most in Australia, but many in New Zealand and Canada. About sixty thousand Micronesians from Palau, FSM and the Marshall Islands live in the United States, Guam and the Marianas (Hezel and Levin 1996; Hezel and Lightfoot 2005; Hezel 2008), over a quarter of all Micronesians from those states, the outcome of little more than two decades of migration. The migration process in Micronesia has quickly become increasingly like that in the South Pacific: a steady outflow, growth of relatively permanent urban communities overseas (beyond student groups), the return flow of remittances and growing interest in migration. Kiribati and Tuvalu have been characterized by migration for much longer, dating back into the nineteenth century, but of contract labour—mainly to Nauru (for employment in the phosphate mine) or into the international shipping industry (for which both countries have training schools)—hence return migration is normal and the impact on national population change much less significant. For smaller islands within all these countries the proportions that have gone overseas are sometimes much higher (e.g. Marshall 2004). By contrast, few Papua New Guineans, Solomon Islanders, i-Kiribati and ni-Vanuatu live overseas, though the contemporary movement towards 'guest workers' in New Zealand and perhaps Australia is beginning to change this. All these crude numbers and trends point to a massive demographic shift towards the metropolitan rim states.

Over time new patterns of increasingly skilled migration have taken migrants beyond more familiar metropolitan rim destinations. Nurses have gone from Fiji to a diversity of global destinations, from Palau and the Marshall Islands to the United Kingdom and the UAE, with active recruitment hastening and emphasizing this process (Connell and Stilwell 2006). Rugby players have gone beyond the 'traditional' destinations of New Zealand and Australia to Japan and the UK. Even newer patterns of emigration have become particularly important since 2003 with a broader structure of migration to the Middle East. Many former Fijian and Tongan soldiers have been employed as security guards for private companies in the major Iraqi cities, and other Fijians are employed in support roles in Kuwait, covering engineering and IT employment (Connell 2006a; Maclellan 2007). New and highly paid overseas employment opportunities are being firmly grasped, even in a threatening security context. So substantial has this new migration become that in 2005 as many as a third of all households in Fiji had at least one overseas migrant—a remarkably high percentage after a relatively short period of engagement in international labour migration (World Bank 2006). These recent events well dramatize the 'outward urge' that has become so powerful in the region. Geographically, economically, socially and politically migration is now more important throughout the Pacific than at any time in the past century.

RATIONALES FOR MIGRATION

While the scale of international migration is affected by fluctuations in the international economy, since the 1980s with accelerating labour demands in metropolitan countries, this has become less crucial as migration has become more significant, more individualistic, more driven by the need for skilled rather than general workers and more able to take advantage of the beachheads established by earlier migrants. The variety of reasons put forward to explain migration in the Pacific sometimes seems interminable and the problems of generalization considerable. Yet migration is largely a response to real and perceived inequalities in socioeconomic opportunities, within and between states, whether in income levels or education and health services. It remains, in different forms, a strategy of moving from a poorer area to a richer one in search of social and economic mobility abroad or at home.

An economic rationale, real or latent, underlies most migration. Simply stated, in Port Vila, one important reason was '*long winim smal vatu from no gat rod long winim vatu long aelan* (to earn a little money since there's no way to earn money on the home island)' (Mitchell 2000: 192). For many that is reason enough, yet four key attractions diversify rationales for migration: 'education, employment, entertainment and excitement' (Marshall 2004: 34). Social influences are important, especially in terms of access to education, but are often a function of economic issues. Politics may also be critical. In Fiji, migration was not only of ethnic Indians, arguably the most affected by the coups, but also of ethnic Fijians, emphasizing how migration could be seen as 'a barometer of fear' of further conflict (Narayan and Smyth 2003). Environmental factors, notably cyclones, have similarly influenced migration, while global warming poses a future threat. In Tuvalu, concerns are such that emigration has already occurred in anticipation of new difficulties to follow (Connell 2003b, 2006a). Expectations have risen over what constitutes a satisfactory standard of living, a desirable occupation and a suitable mix of accessible services and amenities. Employment crises, growing populations, inflation, static (or even falling) commodity prices and the declining availability of land in some areas slowly increase the gap between expectation and reality, at the same time as it becomes more visible. Growing inequalities, coupled with rising expectations, are stimuli for migration. In most places earning power is increasingly concentrated within urban bureaucracies while the absence of developed state mechanisms (such as progressive taxation, unemployment benefits and pension schemes) for affecting transfers of income, minimizes redistribution towards rural areas other than through personal remittances. Experiences and perceptions of the wider world, its values and its material rewards further underlie the migratory experience.

Much tertiary education is undertaken outside the home country, especially in the smaller states where there is limited national training capacity, a factor widely contributing to emigration (e.g. Workman et al. 1981), whilst health referrals may also lead to migration. Moreover, the international movement of students 'represents the internationalization of knowledge, and is arguably the most effective vehicle for creating a global migratory elite' (Koser and Salt 1997: 294). In the Pacific this has been a critical, pump-priming element of the substantial subsequent brain drain (Chapter 4).

Opportunities for migration are greatly valued, freedom of international movement has a high priority and in some contexts fertility may even have risen to enable greater access to migration opportunities. This is exemplified at the household level in Tuvalu, where parents hope to produce remittance earners and most feel that this necessitates having more than one son (since relatively few women migrate overseas). As one woman said of her only son: 'One is not enough. If he goes away to work, there is no one to look after me here. If he stays and cares for me, no one earns any money overseas'. Another woman recognised that her husband had been correct to insist that they needed more children: 'he said that if we had many children we might have a smart one who could go on to high school and get good work. He will be our road to money and to imported goods' (quoted in Chambers and Chambers 2001: 182–184). While economic factors may be at the core of migration, at household and national levels migration occurs within a cultural context where duty and reciprocity play central roles, and movement is bound up with social and cultural obligations, extending beyond extended families to communities. Conversely, individual migrants may be chosen by extended families with such goals in mind, as in Samoa where individuals are chosen to provide service (*tautua*) to family and the wider community rather than themselves (Macpherson 1994). Where migration has become more difficult, as in Kiribati, those once forced to move away because of limited opportunities have been perceived differently. For migrants from Kiribati who had left their densely populated islands in the 1950s and resettled in the Solomon Islands: 'In earlier days they were called the land-hungry people; they were the unfortunate ones who did not have sufficient land. Now our values have changed. Settling overseas, beyond the oceans of our islands, is something to be sought after . . . So now many consider them, the resettled ones, the fortunate ones and they consider us to be the unfortunate ones' (Schutz and Tenten 1979: 127). Such perceptions have become stronger. Migration is an increasingly attractive option.

Migration decisions are usually shaped within family contexts, as migrants leave to meet family expectations, including financial support for kin. Migration has rarely been an individual decision to meet individual goals, nor has it been dictated by national interests (except perhaps in Kiribati and Tuvalu), but is directed at improving the living standards of those who remain at home and the lifestyle and incomes of the migrants and their families. In Tonga 'there are few opportunities for socioeconomic advancement . . . and migration is perceived as the only solution' (Lee 2004: 135). Migration from Samoa was simply 'to seek wealth for all' (Muliaina 2001: 25). Consequently 'families deliberate carefully about which members would be most likely to do well overseas and be reliable in sending remittances' (Gailey 1992: 465; Cowling 1990). Through this process, extended households, as in Tonga, have transformed themselves into 'transnational corporations of kin' which may strategically allocate family labour to local and overseas destinations to maximize income opportunities, minimize risk and benefit from resultant remittance flows (Marcus 1981). To an even greater extent than for internal migration (where health, education and social reasons explain some part of migration) international migration is more evidently an economic phenomenon.

Developing this notion, Bertram has suggested that the extended households of migrants are characterized 'by remittance transfers among various component parts of the "transnational corporations of kin" which direct the allocation of each island's family labour around the regional economy' (1986: 820), and in so doing not only help to maintain these family and communal networks but even enlarge their social fields of interaction, incorporating them into multilocal networks of support and empowerment. For households in Samoa

> having young wage earners abroad diversified families' earnings streams and reduced their dependence on high-risk activities. Having family members in several locations abroad diversified earning sources and reduced risk levels still further. . . . Families, using intelligence from migrants abroad, periodically surveyed risks and returns in various enclaves and encouraged others abroad to relocate in places in which returns were found to be higher and risks lower . . . If this analysis depicts Samoans as calculative and instrumental, it is because in relation to risk and return they are necessarily so . . . [as] risks and returns available in various places were formally canvassed and modeled by families. (Macpherson 2004: 168)

While this form of household consensus certainly occurs, and demonstrates the significance of access to the migration–remittances nexus, families are not always in agreement about their economic aims and functions, but also exhibit conflict and tensions (Lee 2004: 136; Chapter 6). Moreover, remittances are becoming individualized, so that the idea of collective choice and decision-making within a transnational community of kin is gradually becoming less valid (James 1991; Lee 2003). Conflicts over the use of remittances emphasize, rather than downplay, their role and point to the continued significance of an economic rationale for migration.

A CULTURE OF MIGRATION

Migration is now embedded in Pacific life as never before. Epic voyages of exploration and settlement and ancient trading cycles have given way to more prosaic but equally long-distance journeys to new kinds of work. Not only are most countries involved but migration is now more likely to be permanent (even if never the intention), to be invaluable for national and household economies within the Pacific and to have shaped attitudes to education, employment and leisure. Particularly for the Polynesian states such a high proportion of ethnic Polynesians are overseas that the balance of life has shifted towards the metropolitan states and migrants there are key influences on subsequent migration patterns. In a transnational world, contact between migrants and those at home is easier than ever before. Cultures and economies of migration are shaped by the stories, advice and experiences of those who have gone before.

This is most dramatically exemplified in Niue, where the population has fast dwindled with visual, social, psychological and epistemological outcomes (Connell 2008b). Here and elsewhere, especially where nationals are also citizens (or an equivalent in migration rights) of distant metropolitan states, a culture of migration has emerged where migration is pervasive and based on historical precedents, with decisions to migrate part of everyday experiences and migration widely accepted as an appropriate and legitimate means to economic and social well-being (Kandel and Massey 2002; Cohen 2004). Migration has become neither rupture nor discontinuity in personal and household experiences, but an integral part of Pacific life, and normative, where people expect to live and work overseas at some point in their lives, though they also expect never to 'abandon' home or their kin there.

Migration in most islands is an inescapable and pervasive part of life. It has been a part of development plans; through remittances it finances national and household economies. It pervades local cultures, which in turn are shaped by it; as population gravity shifts overseas, a television culture is emplaced and international and local mobility have made islands small. It generates costs and benefits, hope and despair—often simultaneously—at individual, household and national levels. Folk heroes, now regularly observed on local television, such as the rugby players Jonah Lomu and Lote Tuqiri, are constant reminders that success can be achieved elsewhere. As a Niuean pointed out: 'in the old days Niue was a big island—going to town was an exciting adventure—now it is nothing'. Action is now elsewhere. More than in almost any other part of the world migration is 'deeply engrained into the repertoire of people's behavior, and values associated with migration become part of the community's values' (Massey at al. 1998: 47). International migration is thus viewed in different dimensions as a kind of 'safety valve', reducing pressures on national governments to provide employment opportunities and welfare services, and on households to be self-reliant. The ensuing paradox is well illustrated in the observations of Kuini Lutua, the General Secretary of the Fiji Nursing Association (FNA):

> Global economic changes and the law of supply and demand for skilled health professions is [sic] affecting the retention of skilled health workers in countries that can ill afford losing such category of health personnel. For Fiji and other small Pacific island countries in the region sending off a relative for a job overseas is considered a great privilege because of the returns that relatives back home would get from such moves. (2002: 1)

This 'safety valve' effect, and even 'privilege', has resulted in steady and domestically unimpeded outmigration.

In Polynesia particularly the significance of migration is not new. Interest in migration has long been such that in Samoa, when prospects for emigration were particularly poor at the start of the 1980s, the 'broken dreams' of potential migrants contributed to a significant rise in youth suicide (Macpherson and Macpherson 1987). At a national level the economic future of several states partly hinges on the continued flow of remittances, and hence on some continuity of migration (Ahlburg 1991; Connell and Brown 2005; World Bank 2006). The possibility of blocked migration in the future, a situation ever present in public debate (Macpherson 1992; Shankman 1993), emphasizes the potential problem of a high rate of natural increase, especially since a now established 'culture of migration' embraces a contemporary situation where emigration is normal, expected and anticipated, and is an important element in household and national social and economic systems. It is in this broad context that skilled migration occurs.

TOWARDS SKILLED MIGRATION

In the Pacific it has not necessarily been the most educated who migrate first, given the early demand for factory labour, but there has been a steady shift towards skilled migrants as migration policies in recipient countries have become more selective. Broad migration opportunities in metropolitan states have declined, and migration policies in metropolitan states have increasingly targeted skilled migrants, rather than family reunions. Consequently both illegal migration and the growing dominance of skilled migration have occurred. Fiji and several other island states are now seen in Australia as 'high-risk' states because of the extent of overstaying, while there are many illegal Fijian and other overstayers in the United States (e.g. Scott 2003) and New Zealand. The growing shortage of skilled workers has also contributed to increased intra-Pacific migration with workers migrating to countries offering better work conditions and salaries, such as Fijian nurses and teachers migrating to the Marshall Islands and Palau, and tourism workers moving to the Cook Islands.

Male migration preceded female or family migration from most islands. In many cases, families now migrate as units, at least to the metropolitan rim, often as skilled migrants on the basis of one spouse's qualifications. Some specific occupational categories are either male or female dominated. For instance, Fijian women have migrated as nurses, domestic helpers and caregivers while Fijian men have moved overseas as soldiers, tourism workers, police, pilots and security guards. More than two thousand ethnic Fijian women, many undocumented, work as caregivers in the United States, earning and remitting significant sums (Connell and Voigt-Graf 2006: 53). Skills are not necessarily based on educational qualifications; rugby in Fiji, Samoa and Tonga is seen as a 'ticket out of poverty'. More generally the demand for service sector workers, in areas from domestic service to tourism, IT and health has shifted the balance in favour of women.

It is impossible to identify the extent to which SHWs are a significant and rising proportion of either emigrants from Pacific island states, or of immigrants from island states to metropolitan states, since migration data are unavailable: part of a general unwillingness of both sending and receiving countries to acknowledge flows of skilled labour. There are, however, clear indications that SHWs are a proportion of immigrants from Pacific island states to metropolitan states. Each of the principal destinations for SHWs—the United States, Australia and New Zealand—have the acquisition of permanent skilled migrants as one of the objectives of their immigration policies and are competitors in seeking to attract skilled migrants (Cobb-Clark and Connelly 1997). New Zealand at least has actively recruited SHWs in the Pacific island states, notably in Fiji. From the late 1990s there has been recruitment from such distant nations as the United Kingdom, UAE, Bermuda and South Africa. As demand has intensified, Pacific island nurses, usually entering the lower levels of the 'global health care chain', have migrated much greater distances and increasingly as individuals.

Migration of skilled workers began in the prelude to independence, mainly in the 1970s, at least in Polynesia and Fiji, and expanded in the post-colonial era, even as newly or almost independent Pacific island states were developing indigenous workforces to replace colonial staff. Though most early migration was of unskilled workers, it also included a small number of skilled workers, significant because there were so few of them. As early as 1971 the costs of the skill drain from Fiji had already been recognised:

> There are long gestation periods involved in many types of professional, technical and vocational skill training and in the short run the output of these skills cannot be radically changed. In the next few years, despite special and temporary government measures to circumvent or mitigate the problems, the combination of the emigration of skilled and trained manpower, inadequate training facilities and insufficient numbers of skilled people estimated to be in the pipeline . . . will together contribute to a deterioration of the skilled manpower situation with most serious shortages occurring in the supply of technicians and qualified tradesmen. (Ward 1971: 236)

For some states this migration pointed to what was increasingly perceived as a brain drain, first recognised in Fiji (Ward 1971; Bartsch 1974). Occasionally the 'drain' was dramatic. The Cook Islands, for example, lost more than half its vocationally qualified population between 1996 and the end of the century, following externally imposed domestic restructuring after the national economy collapsed (Connell 2005). In the case of migration of Tongans and Samoans to the United States alone, not the most important destination for either state, and certainly not in the 1980s, '[e]migration results in the permanent loss of young educated skilled labour from the Pacific island nations. Skilled labour is in short supply and emigration probably hinders development' (Ahlburg and Levin 1990: 84). The education and skill bias in migration is widespread. As early as 1974 a special study was commissioned on the skill drain from Fiji, which made recommendations for the provision of more appropriate and cheaper training courses in

Fiji that would not meet international criteria, the introduction of bonding for students, the payment of an 'emigration tax' and the repayment of the public costs of post-primary education (Bartsch 1974: 7). Other than bonding, these suggestions were generally not put into practice.

By then private medical students from Fiji and Samoa were already being educated abroad and usually not returning, while government scholarships were given to students whose qualifications 'would not be needed at home'; yet overall, 'although the brain drain is not unknown, emigration by higher level manpower already established in the islands is not generally regarded as a cause for concern' (Bartsch 1973: 10, 88). The reasons for students not returning to Pacific states were that 'the studies may have taken several years at an impressionable age and that they have married while there' (Bartsch 1973: 10, chap. 6). This was the first formal acknowledgement that a selective movement was becoming more than a trickle. Indeed, fifteen years later it constituted 'a very substantial skill and brain drain' (Connell 1987b: 24). Such trends were then only incipient elsewhere.

Skilled migration itself was selective. In the years after independence Indo-Fijians felt themselves 'strangers in their own land' and they were the vast majority of migrants. Between the 1960s and the end of the 1980s Fiji lost around one hundred thousand citizens overseas, almost 30 percent of them in the two post-coup years 1987–1989, after a brief period in the mid-1980s when Fiji was more or less self-reliant in health workers. Within a year of the coups, about a third of the health workforce had emigrated, involving ancillary and nursing staff and including 160 doctors, almost all of whom were Indo-Fijians (Lander and Miles 1992: 29). Between 1987 and 1996 some 205 doctors resigned, a 65 percent turnover (Azam 1996). Almost all (78 percent) of those who then resigned were Indo-Fijian, but in the wake of the coups a new movement of Fijians became evident. Between 1984 and 1994 Fiji lost 586 doctors through emigration (although proportionately the decline was less than it was for teachers). Parallel changes were going on in other parts of the health sector although these were less dramatic because of the small numbers in particular categories. The number of dentists fell from sixty-seven in 1986 to forty-eight by the end of the following year (the year of the coups) and to forty in 1994 (Gani 1999: 99). Here too the majority of the skilled professionals were Indo-Fijians. The same pattern of skilled migration continued and in 1999 the MOH launched its own inquiry into the situation. It was then estimated that 78 percent of the doctors who had resigned in the previous thirteen years had gone overseas, while the others had moved into the private sector. Rural areas had been particularly disadvantaged. In the present century the extent of migration has barely diminished, with one estimate of the equivalent of 65 percent of Fiji's output of graduate nurses migrating each year (Robertson 2006: 33). Lack of documentation of attrition or migration rates in any Pacific state means that such estimates are largely anecdotal, but not necessarily inaccurate.

In other Pacific island states migration of SHWs was generally later and less dramatic (not being a response to coups), with a more gradual impact on health systems, and badly documented. Both Tonga and Samoa experienced the steady loss of SHWs from the 1980s. In Tonga, even in the early years of emigration, between 1950 and 1975, migration tended to be of the relatively skilled. Typical occupations 'for men were the practice of medicine, teaching, administration, trader and the Christian Ministry, with nursing and teaching favoured for women' (Cowling 1990: 198). Tongan doctors 'have sought and taken positions overseas where better terms and conditions of service are offered' (World Bank 1994: 226). Rather later 'continued emigration of qualified and experienced medical personnel has implications for maintenance of both standards and education' (ADB 2002a: xix). A 1995 survey revealed that fourteen doctors had left the Tongan health system in the previous decade. One had retired; at least eight of the others had moved overseas. By then some five doctors were working in Australia, three were in New Zealand, two in Fiji, one in Samoa and two were unemployed in the United States. Several had failed to return from overseas training and had been dismissed from the health service (Wolfgramm 1995). The primary cause of emigration was economic, relating to salary levels, but the location and interests of spouses and other extended family members were highly influential. In the case of Tongan doctors working in Australia, the key influences were starting salaries (with doctors arguing that it was unfair for them to start on similar salaries to others, such as accountants, whose training was much shorter) and the unavailability of adequate medical equipment in Tongan hospitals, which made work more risky and resulted in blame being attached to the doctors for inadequate performance (Fisi'iahi 2001). Roughly the same was also true within dentistry; one new dentist, recently returned from overseas training, commented:

> The main obstacle that we are faced with at the clinic is that we are under-staffed because every day the clinic is packed with people, and there are not enough resources. Dental equipment is very expensive so we are just doing what we can with what we have. (Quoted in *Matangi Tonga* 17, no. 3 [November 2002]: 38)

He went on to say that if he had no luck finding a wife in Tonga within three years 'he would pursue further work experience or studies overseas' (ibid.), a measure of the manner in which migration is integral to Tongan life. By 2004 the loss of nurses had also become evident; though the official nursing vacancy rate in Tonga was just 5 percent, seventy vacancies out of an establishment of 404 were filled by students, suggesting a real vacancy rate of about 20 percent. During that year alone nurses were resigning at the rate of about one per month.

In Samoa it was delicately argued at the start of the 1990s that:

> Many new graduates have not been satisfied with salaries offered and have acquired more remunerative positions elsewhere. According to one 1992 estimate, some 50 per cent of medical graduates migrated over the period 1958–1991 with 80 per cent of this loss occurring since 1980. (Cited in World Bank 1994: 322)

Similar problems of retention were evident for other skilled workers, including pharmacists and dentists (and outside the health sector), and simply assumed to be 'due to salary levels offered by the government relative to alternative employment opportunities in the region and rim countries' (World Bank 1994: 323–324). Somewhat later the World Bank further recorded:

> One of the chief problems of the health system is the shortage of trained health personnel—especially doctors, specialist nurses, pharmacists, laboratory technicians—positions that require extensive education. . .. Poor management, weak supervision and lack of satisfactory training further compounds this problem. Low public salaries make it difficult for Samoa to retain trained medical staff. Many staff move to the private sector or emigrate in search of higher remuneration. Attrition is particularly damaging when public funds are used to train personnel who later leave the public sector. (World Bank 1998: 18)

At that time over 40 percent of the doctors who remained in the public sector were above retirement age. By the late 1990s there was also a more general shortage of nurses, then attributed to inadequate wages compared with those that were available overseas (Samoa 2000). Since then this situation has not improved.

There has been a similar but steady migration of health workers from both the Cook Islands and Niue, enhanced and eased by their being citizens of New Zealand, often undertaking training courses there and having a preponderance of relatives there. In both states this has led to a shortage of doctors at different times from the 1980s onwards—and especially in the Cook Islands from the mid-1990s. While both states have tended to be more or less self-sufficient and reasonably well supplied with nurses, intermittent shortages have also occurred for other SHWs where the actual numbers required are small.

In Kiribati, as in parts of Melanesia, the first significant losses were of expatriates. The number of doctors declined in the 1980s, as British doctors left after independence, and the government pursued a policy of localization (Kienene 1993: 251). Though the impact of this loss was partly offset by United Nations volunteers, by the early 1990s the shortage of skilled personnel was well evident (Chapter 6) and migration was a prominent cause:

> Doctors are also leaving the country in search of better opportunities. Indeed opting to work elsewhere is not new to the medical profession in Kiribati. This has been going on since the 1960s for various reasons such as: family links (intermarriage with non-Kiribati spouses), monetary reasons and personal problems. Indeed, the resignation rate amongst doctors is higher than any other job in the country. This is probably due to the professional nature of the job—doctors are marketable in other countries. It was in 1990 that the greatest single exodus of Kiribati doctors occurred. They all went to work in other Pacific countries: Papua New Guinea, Solomon Islands and Marshall Islands. Such a sudden mass resignation was unheard of in the history of health care in Kiribati and was quite alarming for many in the community, especially because among the six doctors who left were the country's only two surgeons. (Kienene 1993: 254)

In 1996, three i-Kiribati doctors did not return to Kiribati after completing their training in New Zealand, and two others were working in Fiji, two in American Samoa and two in Nauru. Though these numbers are tiny they were a significant proportion of all i-Kiribati doctors and of all i-Kiribati emigrants. Kiribati has continued to experience a shortage of doctors, nurses and other SHWs, estimated in mid-2002 to be about 10 percent of requirements (Easthope 2002). There has been some recent improvement, a combination of improved training and the success of bonding in encouraging the return of those educated overseas.

Even the Marshall Islands and Palau, with fewer indigenous SHWs, have not escaped their emigration. Palau has lost many students following training in the United States and has had a long-term shortage of SHWs. Local frustrations over wages and conditions enabled some recruitment of Marshallese nurses to the United States. In 2001 and early 2002, a Marshallese man working for a company based in the United States recruited four nurses for old-persons homes in the United States, none of whom returned. He was prevented from further entry into the hospital, precluding direct recruitment, but the American company then recruited potential nursing students directly from high school. The same company was also recruiting nurses from Pohnpei (FSM), and probably elsewhere in the region. Even retaining the small number of existing skilled nurses has thus proved difficult enough.

Typical of other Melanesian states (except Fiji) Vanuatu has lost few nurses, though a handful have gone to New Caledonia and the Cook Islands, but a steady trickle of doctors have gone elsewhere. While Fiji may be unique in having experienced coups it is not the only island state to have experienced political problems with negative health outcomes. The Solomon Islands experienced considerable localized violence at the turn of the century, mainly around the capital Honiara. This severely affected the economy, devastated welfare services, including the health care system, which had largely broken down by the end of 2002, and led to the emigration of many skilled workers who were able to move. Two expatriate doctors in the Cook Islands, both of whom had moved there in 2001, were from the Solomon Islands; ironically one of these stated, 'I took up medicine because there were not many doctors in the part of the Solomons I came from, so it was a challenge for me, but I wished to help the people'. As the experience of migration to the Cook Islands from the Solomon Islands illustrates, alongside recruiting within the region (for example, by the Marshall Islands and Palau), some health care systems have gained at the expense of others in the region.

The migration of SHWs (and other skilled workers) has long been part of the process of emigration, but has accelerated since the 1990s. Specialists are particularly likely to migrate (Chapter 6). Of some twenty-five graduates of the FScM who went on to obtain fellowships though the Royal Australasian College of Surgeons in the 1980s and 1990s, only one is known to have returned to practice in a Pacific island state (Oman 2007: 2–3). Similarly, from a sample of sixty-six Fijian doctors who had undertaken specialist training between 1996 and 2004 some thirty-two were in the public sector, but the majority were either in private practice or overseas (Oman 2007: 79). Despite an informal agreement between countries in the region not to encourage the migration of health personnel from nearby island states, this has been practiced for some time. At least three Fijian doctors worked in American Samoa in 2004, and many other islander doctors work in different Pacific states. The Marshall Islands, Palau and Nauru have long recruited Fijian nurses, who often went on contracts of several years, for the experience and because of substantially greater incomes; in Marshall Islands the average nursing salary is about three times that in Fiji. Palau more recently began to recruit Fijian nurses as did New Zealand. In 1999 a newspaper article entitled 'Nurses chase New Zealand jobs' (*Fiji Times*, 3 June 1999) stated that more than seventy nurses had attended specially established interviews designed to attract nurses to New Zealand. The United Kingdom was recruiting Fijian clinical nurses at the same time, and the UAE joined in at about the same time. Not only has the migration of SHWs grown steadily as individuals have made particular decisions about migration, but active recruitment has accentuated this trend. A greater and more visible recruitment of Fijian nurses occurred at a time when it had become more difficult to retain nurses because of dissatisfactions with wages, conditions of employment and political circumstances.

Even estimating the number of skilled workers overseas is impossible. Yet there are clues. By the 1990s at least ten Samoan doctors were in private practice in New Zealand alongside others in private hospitals (Liki 1994: 96), a similar number were in American Samoa and others were elsewhere. More doctors were overseas than working in Samoa. In New Zealand the Niue, Cook Islands, Tongan and Samoan nurses all have registered nursing associations. That of Tonga began in 1984 when twenty-six nurses attended the first meeting, while the 2003 meeting of the Samoan Nurses Association of New Zealand had two hundred people there. But this is the tip of the iceberg. It was estimated in 2002 that there were as many as 127 active Cook Islander nurses in New Zealand, alongside 280 Fijians (mostly Fijian rather than Indo-Fijian), 511 Samoans, 192 Tongans, 75 Niueans and over a hundred others, from Tokelau and elsewhere (Koloto 2003). Even though these figures refer to ethnicity (and not necessarily, therefore, migration) the absolute numbers for all but Fiji are much larger than the number of nurses practicing in the relevant Pacific states. Moreover, there are also substantial numbers from all these states in Australia, the United States, Canada and elsewhere (alongside large numbers of 'inactive' nurses, who may have retired, resigned or taken up other jobs). At least for the Cook Islands, Niue, Tonga and Samoa there were many more nurses overseas than at home. For Niue, Tonga, Samoa (and also Tuvalu) and possibly Fiji, there are at least as many doctors overseas as at home, but no real data to calibrate numerous 'back-of-the-envelope' calculations.

THE OUTWARD URGE

International migration has extremely quickly become of massive contemporary importance through much of the Pacific. Emigration is gradually becoming conspicuous by its presence, as domestic migration has been overshadowed. Once a safety valve for high population densities, migration has now become a safety valve for stagnant economies, political crises and social change. Skilled workers are relatively easily able to migrate, and crises quickly provoke their migration, as they have done in Fiji. Yet, for other than political crises, the consistency in the economic rationale for migration is striking (Chapter 5). Migration has become more complex, with a partial transition from unskilled to skilled workers, globalization has extended the number of destinations and new selectivity has favoured the migration of women. Numbers overseas are necessarily uncertain, as is the extent to which migrants practice high-level skills or move into other employment (Chapter 6), but a distinct brain drain is generally evident. Large concentrations of Pacific islanders are now established in overseas destinations, such as Auckland, Sydney and Honolulu.

So rapid and pervasive has migration been that for half a century there has been a 'culture of migration' emerging in Polynesia and spilling over into the wider Pacific, especially Micronesia. In Fiji, stimulated by a spate of coups, a similar phenomenon has been described as a 'migrant syndrome' (Mohanty and Naidu 2005). Many islands and island states now also experience a shortage of airline pilots, accountants, engineers, IT workers and other skilled groups. In Fiji, alongside SHWs and teachers, accountants, architects, engineers and vets make up almost 50 percent of all skilled migrants, at some social and economic cost (Mohanty and Naidu

2005: 153; Chapter 6). In some smaller states the recent brain drain has been equally worrying; the Cook Islands, for example, lost over more than half its vocationally qualified population in just five years, and even Niue has had to import refrigeration and other engineers from the Philippines because of its losses of human capital to migration (Connell 2008b). Skilled migration is unlikely to decrease, given worsening skilled worker shortages in the 'standard' destinations, and increased shortages in newer, more distant markets.

Although return migration occurs, the volume is always smaller than the flow outwards, notably in Polynesia and Micronesia. A declining commitment to return has been well documented for Samoa (Macpherson 1985, 1994). Limited return is partly due to great differences in income levels, but also to education overseas (for both children and parents), and the loss of certain cultural values, such as linguistic fluency, over generations. In turn this is linked to a gradual shift in the demographic balance, with relatives increasingly likely to be found overseas (see Chapter 6). Interest in migration, and its impacts, has never been greater. How this has come to be so, at least for SHWs, can now be explored.

4 Becoming a Health Worker

> It had always been my intention and dream to be a nurse when I grew up so that I could care for my family and for myself as well. I managed to get work and some training in the United States since, although my father's salary was very low, my uncle in California offered to help by taking me there, putting me through school and later finding a job for me to support my family.
>
> (Thirty-two-year-old Samoan nurse)

Early studies of health workers in the Pacific recognised that migration was primarily related to quality of life issues that involved the employment context (poor working conditions, inadequate facilities, limited opportunities for research or career development), income (particular professional salary structures, costs of living) and a variety of social factors (educational opportunities for children, morale), though not necessarily in that order. A similar range of factors was usually also assumed to account for their migration to capital cities in the region or to take up employment with regional institutions (Naidu 1997; Rotem and Bailey 1999). None of these factors are surprising; they parallel similar conclusions elsewhere and are broadly replicated throughout the Pacific (Chapter 5). However, underlying these immediate influences is an increasingly evident predisposition to migration, and an orientation to it, that begin much earlier than eventual migration in adult life. For many, choosing to become an SHW opened up possibilities of migration that would have been absent in many other occupations. In several small Pacific island states, as people choose to become nurses or doctors (and some other occupations) as a means of migration, their training effectively constitutes the acquisition of human capital directed to acquiring a job overseas.

A vast range of reasons explains why Pacific islanders became health workers. Most had multiple, interlocking reasons, while some had long forgotten what were the critical influences on them; hence, it is neither easy nor particularly useful to produce numerical tables. It is, however, important to assess what for many SHWs is essentially (if sometimes unintentionally) a stage in the migration process. Even before entry into a tertiary institution or the workforce some people seek to become SHWs at least in part, and sometimes primarily, because that provides an obvious means of international migration. In the Pacific as elsewhere nurses were more likely to explicitly indicate that migration was a reason for job choice, whereas for doctors it was implicit. A similar situation has become evident in the Philippines, the Caribbean, India and elsewhere

(Ball 1996; Thomas 2008; Connell 2008c) and appears to have gradually become more universal.

While entering health professions may enable employment overseas it does not guarantee it, especially for nurses, nor is it necessarily sought. Nurses in Vanuatu, the Marshall Islands and Kiribati had qualifications that would not normally be recognised overseas, and none had joined the health profession with the intent of moving overseas. On the other hand, with or without qualifications, citizens of the Cook Islands, Niue, Palau and the Marshall Islands could migrant freely to metropolitan states; hence, becoming an SHW had no necessary bearing on migration, though it would provide a better opportunity for good employment overseas. Becoming an SHW with the objective of migration was thus most common in the larger, independent states.

AN OVERSEAS ORIENTATION?

In Samoa, Tonga and, to a lesser extent, Fiji migration underpinned many decisions to become a health worker, especially for nurses and a range of ancillary workers. In each case this has been relatively recent, both as migration has become more generally significant and as the status of nursing has changed. Until the 1980s nursing in Tonga was considered somewhat menial and 'dirty' and not 'ladylike' compared with teaching (James 2003: 316), which were often the two key options for girls.

> Nursing in Tonga it's like a lower class thing. Like when I was brought up in the 70's and 80's it's not a really a good job to do nursing . . . doing nursing it's like a lower class thing, like you go wiping people's bums . . . It's like you're a filthy person, if you talk about sex, educating people in sex or how women make babies and taking pills. (Quoted in Fusitu'a 2000: 37)

Much the same was true elsewhere in the region, despite a certain glamour also being attached to nursing, centred on uniforms and service (see the following). As nursing (and other professions) became marketable overseas they became valuable and even more respectable. Indeed, in Fiji nursing only became a respectable profession for Indo-Fijian women—rather than an unclean and low-status occupation—when it offered qualifications that could be marketed abroad (Leckie 2000: 78), a situation analogous to that in India (e.g. Thomas 2008).

By the 1980s it was evident not only that becoming an SHW provided upward social mobility—and an income—for many women who might otherwise have been unemployed, but that nursing offered job opportunities outside the Pacific. So prevalent was this new attitude to nursing that in Tonga 'it became a much discussed stereotype'. As one migrant Tongan nurse in Sydney observed:

> When I was in Nursing College we were sort of talking about it . . . it's like a big thing at the time that nurses do their training, then they graduate and then on their three months leave, it's a way of leaving the country. They go on their holiday and they never come back. (Quoted in Fusitu'a 2000: 35)

What was true of nursing was as true of other health professions: 'I became a dentist basically to get out of the country'. Kin usually supported these choices because such jobs were prestigious, remittances would follow and newer migration opportunities might ensue. In Tonga at least, where there is no problem recruiting nurses, people do not enter for the profession but simply because 'it is a job opportunity, where they can go [overseas] on scholarship, and not come back [hence] their hearts are not in it'. Yet many do not migrate and remain in the profession.

While individuals stressed their own strategic choices, in most cases parents specifically encouraged their children to enter the profession for the same reason, while even teachers promoted similar themes:

> I never forget one of the teachers at home saying to us 'You know, if you work in another job, like teaching or something, it's really hard to get a job but if you do nursing, wherever you go you get a job', so I never forgot that. When I arrived here [Sydney] I just asked for a job in a nursing home. (Quoted in Fusitu'a 2000: 35)

This emphasis on the positive attributes of migration, even from within the training institutions that were developing national workforces, pointed to the emergence of a second parallel 'culture of migration'.

Whether or not those in the process of becoming SHWs were actively considering migration, and most probably were not, it was clearly understood by all that at the very least 'whether in Australia or Tonga, nursing training translated into accommodation, food and some kind of pay with the possibility of travel' (Fusitu'a 2000: 36), a not unattractive proposition. Ultimately while only a small number of SHWs indicated bluntly that they entered the profession since this was 'a job to get out of the country', about a third of all SHWs in Samoa, Tonga and Fiji had this in mind at the point of becoming an SHW. Employment in the health system thus enables migration while also being an instigator of it. In turn this further suggests both the complexity of migration and, more importantly, its sometimes tangential nature to the health care system. It also explains why nurses especially do not always continue nursing careers after overseas migration, with migration thus constituting both a brain drain and a brain loss (Chapter 6).

EDUCATION, TRAINING AND MOVING AWAY

Both island nations and households invest substantially in education and training. Partly because of migration opportunities exist in most places for a potential career in the health service. Acquiring a scholarship is the primary means of gaining skills, and of gaining early experiences of overseas life. Most SHWs, other than many nurses, have gone overseas for tertiary education and training at some point. Only in Fiji and PNG were doctors, pharmacists and dentists trained within the region (and most had further training overseas), though apart from Niue and Palau all nurses were trained locally. Nurses later developing a specialization or further training also usually went overseas, usually top metropolitan states. Particularly long periods of training sometimes led to prolonged stays overseas, some attrition and the failure of trainees to return, even when bonded. Neither attrition nor migration were as evident when training was in home countries. For smaller states, such as Palau and Niue, where almost all training is overseas the losses are considerable. In Palau:

> Of those students who go into medicine, nursing and allied health fields and successfully complete in the United States, only a handful return home to work. Others remain in the US or its territories for reasons of their own. There are a limited number of Palauan students who choose health and medical fields at any given time. Of those who initially do, many eventually change their education paths to other fields due to inadequate preparation. . .. Also a good number of these students who initially choose medical, nursing and allied health fields have poor study skills and time management skills making it even more difficult for them to succeed. (Tellei and Renguul 2003: 8)

However while many Palauans who train in the United States remain there, those trained in Fiji have invariably returned. Yet, for the same kinds of reasons, in the Marshall Islands and elsewhere, it has proved very difficult to reduce the demand for tertiary education in the United States in favour of more appropriate systems nearer to home, where return is more likely.

Early on, therefore, much migration was for further education and training, posing a 'training conundrum' where it sometimes went beyond the specific needs of particular jobs. Indeed, most people sought to acquire the highest level of skills possible, where the economic gains were greatest, at least partly because that would enable migration. Additional training was eagerly sought after, beyond its local applicability, while many existing SHWs:

> seek opportunities to have their qualifications recognized by professional bodies and colleagues in developed countries, even though many of them are well trained for the roles they occupy in the home countries. Furthermore training and licensing requirements in destination

countries greatly exceed what is needed in their countries of origin. (Pak and Tukuitonga 2006: 34)

Training in the Pacific had become a classic example of the 'diploma disease' (Dore 1976). Wherever training occurs, as in the case of Tongan nurses, an 'important element which has permeated nurse training options in Tonga has been whether the training will be acceptable in New Zealand and Australia rather than [meet] the real needs in Tonga and the Pacific' (World Bank 1994: 227). Raising training levels to meet overseas requirements had previously resulted in a situation where Tongan nurses acquired overseas employment with relative ease. The more that skills are developed the more they cannot easily or willingly be applied in the Pacific, especially in smaller states, where workers needed to be generalist and multi-skilled. Moreover, the more that training occurs overseas, the greater the propensity to become familiar with new places and people and remain there afterwards. Island states have thus tended to lose the 'best and the brightest', the most able who have undergone the most overseas training, acquiring significant and valuable skills of limited local utility (Chapter 6) alongside new social ties. What might otherwise be seen as an almost obsessive demand for training is oriented to the possibility of future migration, and links in to a medical 'culture of migration'. Whether migration occurs or not, the acquisition of experience and sophisticated skills at home or overseas keeps dreams and options alive.

THE MEDICAL CULTURE OF MIGRATION

Implicit in wide-ranging discontent with conditions in Pacific hospitals and health centres (Chapter 5) is that superior facilities lay elsewhere. For some SHWs such facilities dominated their own training; others learned of the latest overseas technology from those who had trained or simply travelled abroad. The almost universal desire to experience the best technology and the best working conditions (including colleagues, medicines, buildings and technology) is implicit, and often explicit, in health care. Aiming for high-quality health care demands access to the best modern diagnostic and recuperative technology, and necessarily that is in the metropolitan countries.

There is a widespread assumption that to be the best possible health worker access to the most modern knowledge, equipment and experience in the most sophisticated systems is not just invaluable but essential. Thus, teaching staff at the FScM and other national institutions, as elsewhere, not only did not discourage migration but judged their own success as teachers and the success of their students on whether they were able to practice in the more competitive medical environments of countries like Australia, the United States and the United Kingdom (Hagopian et al. 2005: 1755; Oman 2007: 26). The best students and the best teachers simply assumed that some part of their future lay overseas. Even some doctors who undertook masters programmes at FScM, the highest qualification available in the region, were uncertain about their value, and believed they were a 'lesser' qualification than overseas qualifications. As one graduate stressed: 'our Masters is being [seen as] just an infant Masters compared to a Masters from India or somewhere else' (quoted in Oman 2007: 87). The workplace and tertiary education culture dictated that excellence was elsewhere.

Media coverage that stresses the inefficiencies of national health systems further emphasizes that superior systems are elsewhere. As an Indo-Fijian migrant who had left Fiji in 1975 and mainly worked in anesthesiology in Australia and New Zealand said:

> In my profession we have to keep in contact with large hospitals and teaching hospitals because technology is changing really quickly and you need to be in a large hospital to be able to have access to complicated patients and complicated technology. (*Fiji Times*, 31 January 2008)

Despite local enthusiasm for a more modern world (Connell 2007c), typically embraced by the medical profession, the more exciting and complicated concatenations of modernity assuredly lay elsewhere. That effectively constituted a rationale for migration.

Additional training is eagerly sought after, to upgrade skills and experience new technology (beyond local needs and availability), and also keep in touch with overseas professionals in order to be recognised by professional bodies and colleagues in metropolitan countries. The outcome has further emphasized the 'diploma disease', where education is more to get a job than to do a job, or at least a job in the home country, and where specialized learning may enable promotion to good positions, but not where such qualifications are necessarily useful. Even indirectly, with promotions limited by a simple lack of senior positions, increased training opens up overseas options, while limited resources frustrate attempts to use new skills. Such additional training, part of a qualifications spiral, emphasizes professionalism, and is thus often widely welcomed, while enabling the possibility of future migration.

Social factors may also nurture outwards orientation. In recent years the omnipresence of mainly American television series, such as *ER*, *Chicago Hope* and *Grey's Anatomy*, but with a legacy tracing back to *Dr. Kildare* and *Ben Casey*, offers glimpses of both a technology (and sometimes a lifestyle) that are simply out of reach in the Pacific but may conceivably be present elsewhere:

> In hospital soaps the health care staff are idealized. Wards are never endemically short-staffed, no-one complains about being overwhelmed by paperwork (indeed how often is anyone seen doing paperwork?), the plots rarely depict the frustration of bureaucratic hold-ups, no-one ever

> complains about underfunding or the lack of equipment [or boredom]. The myth that 'medicine cures people' is perpetrated without question. (Danser 2005: 53; see also Akl et al. 2007; Chory-Assad and Tamborini 2001)

Such series are mythical but in the background of the drama is a world of modernity that seems much less fictional and potentially realizable.

To some extent scholarships, training opportunities and overseas orientation may stem from a curative model that perceives doctors and nurses 'as disease fighters (saving individuals) rather than as health promoters (saving communities)' (Finau, Wainoqolo and Cuboni 2004: 123). Postgraduate training even within the Pacific, let alone overseas, was seen by many as 'a stepping-stone to positions overseas' and 'a ticket to get out of the Pacific' (Oman 2007: 105), while once distant lands represented better and accessible lives. Yet even before tertiary training, secondary education is widely seen to provide the human capital that can maximize employment options at home and abroad. Through education, and the social context of education, a more evidently medical culture of migration (but extended into nursing and allied activities) overlays and has become intertwined with an existing, more pervasive culture of migration. Both cultures are nurtured by the presence of overseas kin, social expectations of migration, training possibilities and effectively shared citizenship.

SCHOLARSHIPS

Because of the expense of training for health employment, scholarships have an important role to play, especially in the poorer, smaller countries and for overseas training. In relatively poor countries like Kiribati scholarship provision has been crucial for ensuring a supply of doctors, along with a positive national public image of doctors. The existence of scholarships is a definite attraction for high school students, and is crucial for employment in ancillary activities that are often unknown or poorly understood. Knowledge about more specialized kinds of health work is limited at school and while many individuals sought to be nurses and doctors, familiar concepts to almost everybody, few otherwise sought to take up specialist positions such as pharmacists or lab technicians. In Kiribati, for example, none of four SHWs in ancillary areas (pharmacy, radiography, lab supervision and dentistry) had wanted to work in their particular fields and two did not know what their jobs actually entailed until they arrived in Fiji for training. They began simply because they received scholarships in those areas. Unlike smaller Pacific countries, such as Kiribati, where professions like lab technician and radiographer are virtually unknown to school-leavers, in Fiji the possibilities in these fields are better known and are seen to provide an attractive career option, especially when students receive a scholarship.

Elsewhere most such positions were generally filled through scholarships, often by people who knew relatively little about what the jobs entailed, unless they followed in family footsteps.

Scholarships especially in medicine (and outside Fiji) were almost always for overseas education and training and hence were not only keenly contested, but were a major precursor to subsequent overseas migration. While overseas scholarship recipients have invariably been bonded to return, some have broken bonds, but more frequently have found overseas working and living conditions satisfying, or have established social and marital ties at critical points in the life-course that are vital influences on later migration, often as soon as the bonding period is over.

Availability of scholarships was a major influence on choice of employment. In smaller countries, above all Niue, scholarships were partly a function of national need, and high school students jumped at the opportunity of any scholarship, even if health was not necessarily their own priority. This was true for all groups of health care occupations, and the linkage between jobs and scholarships was even closer where more specialized skills were required, as for example in dentistry, or where students had limited knowledge of what was required, such as being a lab technician. While many SHWs had gained scholarships in their preferred field, at least as many had not, again particularly in the smaller states, and even getting their first choice was not necessarily straightforward: 'I got a scholarship because the Minister of Health at the time was my mother's cousin'. Choice was constrained. 'I wanted to teach but I got a place in nursing school', 'I wanted to be a travel agent, and my parents thought nursing was a dirty job, but it was all that was available'. A Tongan doctor noted 'I wanted to be an engineer or an airline pilot. Actually I still do, but I got a scholarship to New Zealand to study medicine. I had no choice but to return to Tonga to complete my bond, but at least I am helping a very understaffed hospital'.

Ironically but not surprisingly the outcomes have not always been ideal. Some of those who grasped scholarships because they were there, or were steered into health work by national requirements rather than their own aspirations, later recognised they had made a mistake. As a nurse stated in Niue: 'I'm still confused as to whether I want to be a nurse or a teacher'. Students regularly dropped out of courses; fully six of the ten Niuean nurses for whom relevant information was available would have preferred some other form of employment at the time they began their nursing careers, and were relatively unsatisfied in their particular positions. In a more wide-ranging study 'many people on the island expressed a desire to have a different job' (Heyn 2003: 35). This is a particular problem in a very small state with specific needs, few positions and where relatively few scholarships must be carefully allocated. It is very difficult to find the most appropriate, satisfying and remunerative jobs. Consequently, the health workforce does not necessarily emerge from those who know most about it, are most committed to its goals and necessarily best suited to it. The means of selection in the smaller states effectively condemn some people to dissatisfaction, and perhaps to migration or attrition.

ALTRUISM, FAMILY, INCOME AND PRESTIGE

While migration may underpin many decisions to become a health worker, other factors ranged from a stable, secure job and income to the prestige, even glamour, attached to health work. Even where migration influenced becoming a health worker, it was never the only and not often the most important factor.

The rich diversity of reasons for entering health professions is best exemplified by two large groups of Fijian nurses, who are typical of the broader context, from the capital city, Suva, and Labasa, the main town on the second largest island. Fully half of the sixty-four Fijian nurses interviewed in Suva offered primarily altruistic reasons for deciding to become nurses, while twelve entered the profession in order to care for their families. One nurse specifically entered nursing to 'help the people in my village who were isolated from hospital' although, ironically, she was now living and working in Suva. Seven entered nursing through 'general interest' or because they enjoyed science in high school and five followed another family member into the health profession. Four trained for a source of income and four because they 'admired the uniforms'. Most of the nurses had only ever trained and worked as nurses; only two had changed careers (one being formerly a waitress and the other being a cashier). In Labasa, a similar situation prevailed with comparable diversity. The seventeen nurses there also had numerous reasons for working in the health field. Four became nurses because they 'admired the work done by nurses', 'I just love the nurses' job taking care of people'; one nurse said he had liked nurses since he saw them coming to their village when he was a child. A fourth nurse admired her grandmother who was a nurse. Another nurse wanted to help other people and originally wanted to do missionary work as a nurse. A further four nurses wanted to help their families as well as helping other people: 'I can help the family by becoming a nurse'. One of these four nurses also said that because there were lots of teachers in her family, she wanted to do something different. Another nurse, who said nursing was her 'calling', also wanted to be different from the rest of her family, most of whom were teachers. A male nurse similarly wanted to do something different as 'nursing among males was not common' as well as to help his family. Another nurse 'reluctantly applied and got in' to nursing as it was 'my father's wish'. Finally, four nurses became nurses for the income and job security. One said that she had chosen to go into nursing because student nurses were paid. The other three wanted job security, one explaining that after nursing school one goes directly into a job, unlike other jobs where one finishes studying and then has to apply and wait for a job.

Underpinning most of these reasons, and most had multiple reasons, was the widespread and easily comprehensible aim of helping people, and because there was some degree of prestige and a reasonable salary attached to the profession. Few stressed the significance of migration, at least partly because it was not in the forefront of people's minds and lives. Some SHWs had not been initially interested in a health career at all, or knew little about what it might entail. Many nurses were interested 'since childhood' but the specific reasons ranged from 'I always wanted to be a nurse; I admired nurses in their white uniforms' to 'My father was a surgeon and my brother a doctor; I was always interested and challenged by the medical field but really it's in the family'. Within this complexity and diversity there are clear themes, most linked to situations where they could support their families and their families supported them.

Some of the strongest influences on migration are thus only incidentally related to employment, or at least the structure of employment in the country of origin, but much to do with attempts to improve the long-term welfare and status of families. Throughout the Pacific many SHWs entered the health professions less out of a general altruism, or even less a particular interest in medicine, but through recognition that this might be a means of maximizing, or at least improving, family incomes and welfare. Some even changed professions to provide family support. A Tongan doctor 'was an accountant but switched to medicine to help my family'. A Samoan became a nurse: 'I grew up and I really didn't want to be nurse. However my brother was the main person who persuaded me so that there would be someone to take care of the family's health. As for me, I was hoping to be a teacher'. The most important reason, given by eight of the nine nurses in the small town of Ba (Fiji), for entering the health profession was to help people, but especially their own families: 'I decided to take up nursing to help my family'. Three had sick relatives, which encouraged them to enter the health system, and four were encouraged to join by family members. One also specified 'the need to have a close relative [working at the hospital] to provide good care'. A nurse in 'Eua (Tonga) noted how nurses were selective over which patients they saw first, indicating that kinship structures, pervasive even in public health systems, were invaluable family supports.

Fully twenty-nine out of thirty-four Samoan nurses stated that the most important reason for them to gain nursing training was to care for members of their families. One explained that, 'as an eldest child I was responsible for the health of my family' and another said, 'my dad has got heart disease so they asked me to be a nurse so that I can care for him'. In a country where family responsibility and duty are important it is unlikely that such nurses would emigrate if they had parents or other family members to care for. Since most of the nurses had large families in Samoa, this also explained their remaining in Samoa even when their wages seemed inadequate. Samoan nurses were also more likely than others to talk in religious terms of 'calling', 'religious commitment' and 'doing God's work'.

Such altruism was more important for many than monetary rewards, with one nurse claiming to have rejected a better job offer because it would limit her services solely to those who could afford it: 'MedCen [private hospital] wanted me but I refused because I know only a few people can afford to come there thus my service too will be limited'. Family support thus spilled over into a general altruism to the wider community.

There was a converse to altruism. Various SHWs were encouraged by parents to join the health sector, sometimes because of the assured government employment and reasonable income and sometimes purely to look after their own needs. One nurse who wanted to be a teacher noted: 'My parents were selfish—only thinking about themselves—for me to look after them'. Others became nurses because they saw this as their responsibility: 'I wanted to help people and earn some money for my family'. Helping the family sometimes meant sacrifice. One thirty-year-old Cook Islands nurse, one of the very few who had never been overseas, indicated:

> I was chosen to be a nurse so that I could stay here and look after the land and my parents while my other brothers and sisters went overseas [but] I would like to go overseas to get more experience in nursing, to work in a more modernised situation because I fear I may lose what I have learned if I stay here, but it's hard to get my family to understand since they chose me to stay and the rest of the family are overseas.

Families were thus making decisions not only about jobs but at least implicitly about the future residence of their children. Decisions to become an SHW were therefore rarely individualistic and sometimes involved extended family meetings and discussions, so that decisions were to some extent collective. Again that was particularly true of nurses and older workers, including men. Thus seven out of eighteen Tongan SHWs in Sydney believed that it had been their own choice, seven more said it was definitely not their own choice and the remainder saw it as being a matter of what alternatives happened to have been available at the time (Fusitu'a 2000). Health workers certainly wanted to help people, but particularly their own families or 'their people'. Often that was broken down to local regions, such as 'my own 'Eua people'. Altruism began and sometimes ended close to home.

The predictability, availability and stability of a job in health were strong influences on choice. This was particularly true for older SHWs, especially nurses, who had entered the profession in the 1960s and 1970s, and for whom few other employment choices existed. As one Fijian nurse expressed it, nursing was a 'childhood interest', but 'in those days'—the 1960s—career choices were limited hence 'nursing was the only option'. Another simply said, reflecting a general perspective, that there 'weren't many employment choices available'. Of two other Fijian nurses, who had entered the profession primarily for the income, one said, 'in those days, only nursing and teaching were available for school-leavers, and my interest was in nursing', being influenced by her mother who was also a nurse. The other explained that 'I needed to look for a job to support myself and help my parents. Nursing was available'. More contemporary employment contexts are much more diverse but, while career choices are more fluid, health employment continues to offer a degree of certainty that is not always evident elsewhere. One nurse pointed out that nursing was a good opportunity because even trainee nurses received wages. Another, who wanted to become a psychologist, said that it was 'easier' to do nursing, and then go to university 'because of money problems' and another explained that while she wanted to do catering, staying in Suva for this training was not easy, and 'at least nursing provided hostels'. Becoming an SHW was secure.

Family traditions were also important. Frequently SHWs had modelled their own lives on those of relatives who had become nurses or doctors. As the New Zealand Minister of Pacific Island Affairs, Winnie Laban, stated to the 2003 New Zealand Samoan Nurses Conference:

> We all come from and are descended from nurses. My grandmother and mother were great nurses. We all have personal stories like mine to celebrate. These nurses were our leaders and healers in our community so that legacy lives on with each and every one of you. Our culture is based on the Samoan values of *alofa, fa'aaloalo,* and *agaga*: love, respect, reciprocity and spirituality. These values are demonstrated through *tautua* service. Add modern nursing practices to these Samoan values that we are born with and learn in our families and communities then you have the right mix to develop wonderful nurses. (2003)

These kinds of 'traditions' of service, no mere rhetoric and common in the region, also reflect the underlying roles of status, income and migration potential, as opposed to the menial drudgery that gave nursing low status. Indeed, it remained not uncommon (though less common than support) for families to discourage employment in the health sector, stressing that nursing particularly was 'dirty' and inappropriate work—somewhat in contrast to the perceived glamour of the uniforms. Such negative perspectives and discouragement were more common in rural and regional areas, where households preferred girls to remain at home and support their families in that way, rather than move to distant towns or countries. Some parents (and, no doubt, workers in other professions) felt that employment in health simply had 'too many responsibilities' for the limited income it generated. In contrast, other nurses pointed out that their parents had not approved of their choice of nursing 'simply because lots of nurses became single mothers'. This too was more likely to be a rural perspective.

While becoming a health worker might directly assist families, earning a good income was the most common form of family support, and a key reason for becoming an SHW.

For Fiji, Tonga and Samoa (where the stated propensity for migration was greatest) some 47 percent of those nurses who had migrated overseas had joined the profession for income reasons compared with only 27 percent of those who were still working in their home country. Thus, those who claimed to have joined the profession because of its income potential were most likely to have migrated, and least likely to have stayed at home (Brown and Connell 2004). Even so, income was clearly important for those who had stayed. For Fijian doctors in Fiji, though multiple reasons were given for entering the profession, seven (out of twenty-four) said that altruism was their main priority, while five said that income was the key factor.

For older nurses especially two other factors tended to be generally important alongside the security and income that came from a health position: the freedom that this represented in a regulated, hierarchical society, and the prestige and status sometimes attached to wearing an impressive uniform. Nurses' colleges offered new freedoms. While prestige was rarely the key reason for choosing a health career, and the lure of a uniform much weaker, it was also rarely trivial and frequently implicit. Family tradition emphasized the prestige involved and doctors especially emphasized the prestige attached to being a doctor. As one Fijian doctor stated: 'Top students go into medicine. Everybody looks up to you'. A Samoan doctor spoke for many in claiming that his family wanted him to be a doctor to 'uplift family status and standing in the community'.

DISINCENTIVES

Where women now have more freedom of choice and nursing may be seen as problematic, it is not always as prestigious or as obvious a choice as in earlier years when fewer alternatives were available. Older attitudes which discouraged nurses from taking up nursing because of the possibility of their becoming 'loose women', or because the job was dirty and demeaning, have been replaced by newer attitudes that emphasize poor wages and other alternatives. Attracting SHWs into nursing in a time of AIDS is not always easy, even in Pacific island states where unemployment is high, and AIDS still insignificant. Only in PNG, where night shifts are feared and can be dangerous, and AIDS levels are high, is recruitment particularly difficult. Knowledge of salaries and conditions are greater disincentives to entry into the health workforce.

In the Marshall Islands discontent over nursing salaries (US$7,000 on graduation) compared with those in other professions, the inability of potential nurses to meet entry requirements (because of low educational standards in local high schools), alongside perceptions of hard work, meant that no Marshallese nurses graduated from the College of the Marshall Islands (CMI) nursing school in 2002, and the school was not running at its full capacity. While there was guaranteed employment for nurses, it was also apparent that 'nursing is one of the few professional jobs that requires working on the graveyard "shift" from midnight to morning' (*Marshall Islands Journal,* 10 May 2002). As the head of the nursing programme at CMI pointed out:

> Numerous academic choices have reduced the number of Marshallese students picking the medical profession as a career choice. This coupled with the low salaries paid by the hospital have both contributed to the current shortage of Marshallese nurses. Students tend to gravitate toward computer sciences, business and other courses. Low salaries are a real disincentive to encouraging Marshallese to go to nursing school and to keeping nurses at home once they've graduated. (*Marshall Islands Journal*, 10 May 2002)

The disincentives to entering the profession are broadly those that have posed problems in more developed countries, but are here replicated in circumstances where youth unemployment is extremely high. Perceptions of hard work and public sector salaries have been even more devastating in Nauru, where phosphate mining brought affluence and disdain for any kind of work, producing a situation where: 'We have produced a generation that has a lack of motivation, a lack of discipline, who don't see the need for education, who can't see the point of spending time in FScM or Fiji School of Nursing to be nurses or doctors'. Consequently 1971 was the last time that the health service had been able to recruit Nauruan nurses (Connell 2006b: 51). All newly hired nurses have long been recruited from Fiji.

Alternative employment opportunities are more attractive. Business exercises more fascination for high school leavers in Vanuatu than health care. In American Samoa few girls are interested in a health career; 'smart girls now want to be lawyers, accountants or in business . . . they want "fast money" in the computer field, they don't want to wait ten years to be a doctor'. And in American Samoa migration to the United States is always possible without any skills. By contrast, in Tonga the fact that three years of nursing training meant that nurses would be recognised in New Zealand 'guaranteed that there was no problem of recruitment'. Recruitment of nurses has been more difficult than other SHWs for several reasons, but increasingly because wages and working conditions are less attractive, as long as there are other roads to migration. More specialized SHWs have also been hard to recruit because of unfamiliarity with such jobs and the need for some science background, further complicated by the small numbers of specialists that were required. Recruiting trainee doctors has only been difficult where educational criteria have proved too challenging.

In Palau, the Marshall Islands, the northern Cook Islands, and probably elsewhere, educational disadvantage reduces the chances of most school-leavers becoming SHWs. This prevents there being an adequate supply of

SHWs, either nationally or regionally (as in the Cook Islands), and emphasizes how becoming an SHW is selective, more easily achieved in urban centres and, in turn, more likely to be advantageous there or overseas.

STARTING OUT

A multitude of factors, similar throughout the region, influence beginning a job or a career in health, from migration, altruism and economic need to the lure and prestige of uniforms—an order, propriety and perhaps even cleanliness absent in other jobs—which remarkably often has been one reason for becoming a nurse. The Cook Islands, amongst others, continues to stress the 'smart working uniform' in its work experience programmes for high school students. At the same time, like employment in the police force, the unusual hours meant it was 'not a job youth naturally grab'. Family pressure and support (motivated by income gains, social needs, status and prestige), and even having sick relatives, especially parents, were of considerable importance. The latter provided direct personal contact with the health profession and the recognition that nurses and doctors were invaluable. Medicine was prestigious, incomes were substantial and employment was inherently attractive. Any stigma attached to nursing was more than counteracted by the possibility of migration. It could then be simply a means to another end. Yet most stressed that their entry into nursing was to help others, a perception that they still valued, and indeed helped to define who they were.

Ironically many people, and especially the more skilled, only became health workers because there were scholarships available. The same scholarships that produced SHWs gave them initial overseas experience and a taste of greater economic and social opportunities that might later become international migration. Equally ironically, though health workers stressed their own altruism—and there was no reason to question the genuineness of those who remained in their home countries—a profession where altruism was so often at the fore (more than in most other professions) was also the one that enabled the greatest prospects of migration.

Education and service were important values for many who became SHWs. At least until the late twentieth century, the 'Nightingale tradition' remained in place, which promoted nursing both as a respectable occupation for 'ladies' and as a regulated middle-class career (Leckie 2000: 78). It offered a step up in the world, where other choices might be vetoed by fathers or husbands. As a Tongan nurse in Australia put it:

> You're under the influence of your parents from when you're born, up to the high school, always everything is tight on you. It's like you live in a shell and there is no experimentation . . . There's no other way out of the house except church and besides that you're just home, just cooking, cleaning the house. (Quoted in Fusitu'a 2000: 44)

Education was excitement enough for some. Becoming an SHW provided individual gains especially for women; sometimes they were straightforward: 'Independence, like to explore the world, have a boyfriend, going out dancing, climb out of the window, do silly things' (quoted in Fusitu'a 2000: 49; Barclay et al. 1998). Moving away from home (usually) to train as a nurse offered negligible supervision, new freedoms of movement, socializing and an autonomy rarely easy to achieve in other contexts, even if that might mean that nurses might be seen by some as irresponsible. Yet it almost never meant the abandonment of duty. Indeed, it led to a reliable and potentially interesting job in the stable public sector.

Workers were supported and usually encouraged by their families, as they needed to be over lengthy training periods that might eventually reap benefits from both employment in health care and migration. Decisions about taking up employment, just as later decisions on migration, were characteristically framed within a family context, especially for women becoming nurses. Independence and education were valuable acquisitions but were not couched in terms of individual aspirations, however much girls might have been attracted by the uniforms, wages and excitement of a career. The materiality and physical nature of nursing itself seems rarely to have influenced decisions to enter the profession.

Households invested in education because training was valuable for a secure career in the public service that provided the flexibility to enable island or metropolitan employment. Acquiring skills could easily be justified in terms of both local needs and individual interests. Such individual interests, extended family aspirations and ensuing migration have created unusually skilled and bureaucratic versions of the Pacific 'transnational corporation of kin'. While that transnational corporation of kin has usually been seen in a geographical sense, with migrants from particular households scattered through different nations, it is also structural, as households seek to place family members in vital arenas of employment. Numerous households have sought to strategically position children in key institutions such as banking, education, the police or army, and the health service: for example, 'My family wanted a nurse since I had older brothers in the police force and Ministry of Transport'. Professional and spatial deployment were carefully combined. Employment in health has become an invaluable means of diversifying, both structurally and spatially, extended family livelihoods across countries and continents. It is scarcely surprising that a propensity to take up employment in health begins early, and that in different ways it epitomizes a dual culture of migration.

5 Leaving Home?

Movers and Stayers

> Coming from a large family my parents encouraged me to be a nurse when I grew up so that I could care for the whole family's health. What I like most about this job is helping the people of Samoa. I don't want to change jobs, and waste my experience, since this is the best way to show you love and care for people.
>
> (Thirty-two-year-old Samoan nurse)

Underlying most migration moves are substantial differences in development between places within and beyond the Pacific region. Centred on economic circumstances, but strongly influenced by a constellation of social, political and cultural factors, the migration rationale of SHWs in the Pacific varies only subtly between states and social groups. Where migration has been common in the recent past it is simply expected that others will avail themselves of the same opportunities. Indeed SHWs are as sensitive as any others about their rights to be mobile, as noted by Kuini Lutua of the FNA (Chapter 3). Migration poses no technical problems where islanders are also citizens of metropolitan states, as are Niueans, Cook Islanders and effectively most Micronesians, and is much more fluid there. But increasingly, as dual 'cultures of migration' are consolidated, migration has become more widely normative.

Migration of SHWs occurs for a variety of reasons, despite a remarkable global uniformity, partly because of the emergence of a global care chain and demand-driven migration. Such reasons include income, job satisfaction, career opportunities, management and governance, education and training, politics, and social and family reasons (Connell 2008c). The last of these factors is crucial since migrants rarely decide as individuals but are linked into extended kinship groups and benefit from and provide family support. Decisions are invariably complex, and evolve over time towards a particular, sometimes catalytic, moment. Migration is usually constrained in certain ways. Though there are few countries where additional SHWs would not be welcome, even those with skills cannot always easily cross political borders, or move with families. Many skilled migrants take advantage of particular relationships between sending and receiving countries, such as that between New Zealand and Samoa, which allows a fixed number of migrants each year from Samoa, formerly a colonial possession of New Zealand. Migration thus often flows along former colonial lines.

Most migration of SHWs is actually within countries, and almost every country experiences some internal migration, usually from rural to urban areas and from poor regions to richer regions: analogous to the structure of international migration. The outcome too is also often similar: a concentration of the professional workforce in the larger urban areas and scarcity in remote areas, reflecting inevitable economies of scale, the practical and financial difficulties of meeting the diverse needs of remote places and their peoples, and the task of organizing an adequate structure of health care delivery in the face of staff shortages, restructuring and the regular absenteeism, attrition and mobility of personnel.

Migration cannot simply be differentiated into push and pull factors, and the relative values attached to these factors, so that at some point the balance tilts in a particular way and the logical response is migration. Stories of individual migrants, such as Jane and Rosemary (see pp. 111–2 and 142–4), emphasize just how complex migration can be, and how different people (and their kin) balance factors in quite different ways. It is useful to examine the many factors that have influenced migration, and also stability, in the words of Pacific SHWs, not least because there is some consistency of influences however they are ultimately weighted, ignored, or become major irritants and catalysts. Numerous surveys, including the bulk of the present study, have focused on SHWs within Pacific island states, and examined the possibility of future migration, but intentions are not the same as migration; however determined individuals might have been to leave, their decisions remained in the future. Nonetheless their rationalizations are similar to those of SHWs who have migrated, who play a smaller part here, and are as much a guide to future attrition as to future mobility.

AT HOME

Most people never migrate, but remain permanently in their home countries. While migration is increasingly common in the Pacific islands, many obvious reasons mean that people want to stay, and only reluctantly move. It is home—a familiar place and landscape of kin, friends, land and ancestors, of old family and clan histories, of schools, churches and burial grounds, where others speak the same language, have similar values, attitudes and lifestyles. The land, the sea and extended families offer an anchor and a livelihood, however limited and constrictive this may sometimes be. Home poses few surprises and uncertainties.

Certainly not all health workers seek to migrate, even in countries where migration is common. One earlier analysis of why SHWs remained in Fiji, indicated that the two most significant influences were the rather vague 'job satisfaction' and 'lifestyle' (Naidu 1997: 70–71). What this actually meant, and who these factors most influenced, was unrecorded. While some existing predisposition to migration, or at least keeping options open, exists amongst many SHWs and their families (Chapter 4), most enjoyed their work, had no real grievances with the system and found a considerable degree of fulfillment. That fulfillment came partly from being at home with their families and partly from the specific satisfactions of the job.

Inherent in this is a degree of professionalism and pride that comes from treating and curing sick people—and sometimes from treating one's 'own people' especially those who are poor. For many, Christian (and sometimes other) religious convictions underpinned their working lives, offered some resilience to stress and emphasized a sense of duty. A Hindu Indo-Fijian doctor observed: 'For me, doing something for my God is more important than doing for myself . . . I see everything as my duty' (quoted in Oman 2007: 94). Often such influences were explicitly counterpoised to migration; as a Fijian doctor said:

> I believe you can do a lot more in Fiji . . . if I go and work in Australia, they really don't need me; they have so many good people out there that can look after their children, but if I leave here then a lot of people would miss out on my services . . . I suppose I'm needed and that's why it made me want to stay here. (Quoted in Oman 2007: 90)

Indeed the recognition that they were needed, evident in patients' appreciation and that of their colleagues, was a further factor influencing job satisfaction.

The perceptions and attitudes of doctors and nurses in Fiji were broadly typical of those elsewhere. Thus, twelve of the twenty Fijian doctors had no desire to leave Fiji, and as many as eleven wanted to stay, primarily because 'it's home', which for them meant having families and close friends nearby. Similarly, some twenty-six of the sixty-four Suva Fijian nurses had no plans to leave Fiji, mostly because of family, friends and being established in Fiji. Reasons such as having children in school, owning a good house and spouses having good jobs deterred people from wanting to leave. Some people felt strong ties with their homeland and an obligation to stay. As one nurse declared, 'Fiji needs us'. Another would have preferred to move abroad for the experience and chance to earn a better income but her husband wanted to stay in Fiji and she refused to go alone. As she explained: 'I have to be with my family. Money is not everything'. More prosaically many have stayed fearing that their qualifications and competence would not be recognised abroad or because they were simply 'too old' to make radical adjustments to their lives and those of their families: 'Overseas life is very fast. We are too old to cope', 'no one would employ me overseas' and 'I'm an old woman now'. Others were looking after elderly relatives (sometimes the reason why they had embarked on nursing). For a handful there was being 'afraid of the unknown . . . with my age . . . I think it would be difficult to get a job overseas'. Income was not everything: 'my eldest daughter is in Fiji and money is not a priority, I'm happy with my income'. In a similar vein, another nurse said, 'I'm satisfied here. Working overseas the focus is on money but that is not the most important thing. This is a better place for my family'.

Most Palauan nurses similarly wanted to remain in the local health system, especially when close to retirement, and many too were altruistic: 'I generally like this job—helping people, especially sick people', 'It's my country and I work to help my people', well summarized by one twenty-nine-year-old female nurse:

> Well first of all it is my home country and I feel I owe it to the Palauans that I stay and work for them, even though sometimes it gets frustrating but I can cope with it, and of course my family and relatives are here.

One had returned after twenty-five years way 'to be close to relatives and my beloved homeland'. While almost all had some degree of frustration with the system: 'not enough nurses to take care of sick patients', 'low salary and nurses don't show up on time', 'no promotion' and 'high levels of stress', other factors prevailed. Nationalism was also evident elsewhere. Versions of 'I would rather live here because Vanuatu is my home country with all my family members with me and I also like my own customs and cultural way of life' were common, not only in Vanuatu. Few anticipated going elsewhere, and were enthusiastic about their home country: 'the peaceful nature of the place itself', 'the loving caring people of this country', 'it is a paradise place to live in' and 'it's more peaceful than any other countries'. The way of life in Samoa was more important to many than the chance to earn more money abroad with the majority of nurses considering the freedom in Samoa, the low cost of living and low level of crime good reasons to remain. Large numbers of SHWs simply wanted to work for 'my people', on 'my island' or to stay because 'this is my country': certainties and moralities that they felt needed no further explanation.

Duty and even altruism might be inculcated. Several felt a duty to stay and help their people and their country, sometimes because of financial assistance received: 'I was a sponsored student. I have a duty to serve the people of Fiji'. Sometimes this was simply from national pride and a sense of duty: 'the only reason for choosing to be a doctor is to work in Fiji and help my people in Fiji.' One doctor explained, 'I've worked in Melbourne but it seems that you are only doing it for the money. Here, you don't get much money but you feel that you're really helping people.'

Others were constrained by families. One Marshallese had no wish to go because his extended family was there and he was needed to care for his ill mother as all but one of his siblings had left the Marshall Islands to live in the United States. Samoan nurses had strong ties to their home and often felt obliged to remain because of family ties: 'As a Samoan I am responsible for looking after my mother to get more blessings for me and my children.' Another nurse said that it was 'difficult to go with a family' because of the expense and that if she went by herself she would be separating the family, adding that 'overseas it seems that nursing is about money, here it is your call, and it is more than just a job'. Another did not plan to go 'now' because 'I'm still bonded for one more year' and because her husband wanted to study at USP. Husbands, land, business and property ownership, obvious objectives in life for many, were major deterrents to migration. While a sense of public worth plays some part in decisions to stay, and health workers are more easily able to stress this, pragmatism and inertia have crucial roles. Health workers are part of established families where other household members have strong commitments to the home country.

ENJOYING THE JOB

A very large number of SHWs, perhaps more than in other areas of employment, expressed a sense of both altruism and duty about their work: 'I wanted to pay back the Niuean people and reduce the language barrier that is associated with expatriates, since we understand local values and conditions' and 'I like being able to work with and help my own people'. Ubiquitously SHWs had taken up health work to 'help my people' and remained proud of what they could accomplish: 'a special skill I'm doing for them'. Some even sounded like recruitment posters: 'putting in your contribution to the development of this country' and 'build and promote the community and always protect the health of the nation'. While most i-Kiribati doctors were at least mildly interested in working overseas one declared he would definitely not like to move, which he saw as 'selling [his] freedom' since he would prefer to stay and 'save Kiribati'. While this perspective was rarely entirely absent, such altruism may better explain why health workers took up their positions initially, rather than remained there, as such feelings do not necessarily sustain a career.

Nonetheless, what SHWs most liked about their jobs, as so many claimed, was helping and working with their patients, including being able 'to meet and treat my relatives and friends'. The most positive aspects of their work involved the human contacts involved, such as helping others, meeting new people and working with colleagues. This spilled over into the satisfaction that only a health career could bring: the pleasure in seeing patients recover. 'I like caring for very sick patients and seeing them get well and going home to their families—but hate it when they go down', 'I like being here because I can give something back to the community' or, quite simply, 'I like this job; no other job would be me'. 'The salary's no good but it is good to work with your own people'. While such pleasures are universal, the greater probability of having a social relationship with patients further discouraged migration.

More specialized positions were usually particularly attractive because of the greater responsibilities and increased sense of personal fulfillment: 'midwifery is a special field and I enjoy doing it'. In the larger countries, especially where superior opportunities for further education and training existed, the job itself had additional attractions and benefits. Thus half the Fijian nurses enjoyed learning on the job, 'keeping up with new cases and medications every day', including the benefits of regular seminars and learning from visiting teams. In-service training had a positive effect on morale, alongside its intrinsic value. Another nurse enjoyed teaching and supervising the new nursing graduates. Diverse challenges, training possibilities, helping patients and working effectively with colleagues were what most nurses enjoyed. Personal contacts, a good working environment and being able to learn on the job were as important. A range of factors from being with family, age, having a sense of dedication and a challenging and interesting job were central to SHWs staying at home. Though all these factors had not discouraged others from leaving, their absence increased the probability.

INCOME

Just as being at home with family and the social and professional satisfactions of health employment were key deterrents to migration so a rather larger cluster of factors were key influences on migration. None were individually enough to stimulate migration, which was normally the outcome of many factors. However, broad income differentials have been the major influence in almost every study undertaken of the migration of health workers, in every developing country context and time period (Connell 2008c). In Pacific island states income was a key influence on decisions to join the health profession (Chapter 4); hence, it is not surprising that it also constituted a reason for leaving it. Income differences between countries have become increasingly well known and in some cases are vividly evident: salaries of SHWs in American Samoa may be up to ten times those of workers in comparable positions in Samoa less than a hundred kilometres away. In the midst of the 2005 Fijian nurses strike, the *Fiji Times*, under the heading 'Why they're running away', noted that the starting salary of nurses in Fiji was F$10,000 compared with F$32–34,000 in New Zealand, F$44,000 in Australia, F$45–48,000 in the UK and F$40,000 in Dubai (7 August 2005). Similar discrepancies have prompted other movements. Almost as frequently, working conditions have been linked to income as a second major influence, but one which also accounts for attrition.

For contract migration within or beyond the region, incomes are particularly significant, at least in part because the benefits from going to a metropolitan state, including going with family, superior education, and wide-ranging social amenities are scarcely evident. Every one of a group of fifteen Fijian nurses on two-year contracts in the Marshall Islands had moved for superior incomes more than double those at home (Rokoduru 2008), though invariably other factors—the cultural experience, different and more modern technology or an escape from domestic tension—were also attractions.

Throughout Pacific island states wages and salaries are widely seen as inadequate, while the number of strikes in various states in the 2000s, particularly in Fiji and Samoa (see the following), is some testimony to the extent of dissatisfaction. SHWs are not particularly mercenary but income is an obvious metaphor for various opportunities foregone or overseas, a means of realizing these opportunities and an explanation for migration that makes perfect sense. Two thirds of all nurses and almost half (46 percent) of all doctors were primarily motivated to migrate for income reasons, a conclusion that is common across all Pacific countries. The importance of income, whether absolute or relative, cannot be underestimated.Past migrations had a similar rationale, while earlier surveys in the region have attached even more importance to income. In 1996 a group of Fijian doctors who intended to resign pointed to the main reasons as low salary (55 percent), poor working conditions (41 percent) and lack of postgraduate training (27 percent) with most of the Indo-Fijians intending to move abroad and the Fijians into private practice. Of rather lesser significance were a somewhat nebulous 'need' to migrate (18 percent), job dissatisfaction (14 percent), poor on-call allowance (9 percent) and the lack of malpractice insurance (5 percent) (Naidu 1997). A slightly later survey in Fiji in 2000, conducted by the Fijian Nurses Association, found that for as many as 88 percent of nurses the key influence on migration was higher wages (Leweniqila, Camaivuna and Dokoni 2000). Economic issues are paramount.

The higher the wages in the home country the less the probability of migration, irrespective of income differentials between countries. Doctors were therefore least likely to wish to migrate, and nurses the most likely, while ancillary workers were in an intermediate category. There is an even greater probability, at least in Fiji, that doctors in the private sector would not migrate because of higher salaries and superior working conditions. However, doctors do not necessarily move into the private sector because of the higher wages there. In Fiji doctors moved from the public sector to the private sector because working conditions interfered with family life, they were frustrated with disruptive schedules and bureaucratic ineptitude which limited their autonomy and gave them a sense they were not valued (Oman 2007: 130). Doctors tended to compare their salaries with those of other skilled workers in their home countries and were relatively satisfied. However some SHWs emphasized that they made a particular contribution to society and were not adequately rewarded for that. A Kiribati doctor complained that the wages of doctors, in comparison with other workers, did not reflect the extensive education they had undertaken and the great responsibility they took upon themselves in looking after people's lives: 'doctors offer too much and get little in return'. Various doctors and others felt they were unacknowledged for the time and effort they had put into their nationally important work.

Tongan nurses had a greater propensity to migrate than Samoan nurses, partly because the Tongans earned less than the mean Tongan income whereas Samoans earned more than the mean Samoan income, although in real terms their earnings were about the same and their gains from migration would also have been about the same (Brown and Connell 2004, 2006). The relative income position of nurses (and other health workers) within their home countries—the basic national salary structure—is a critical influence on migration. Every one of the twenty-six out of sixty-four Suva Fijian nurses who had considered working abroad at some stage in the future listed the chance to earn higher wages and get a better job as the main reason for considering migration. In different ways and at different scales, migration demonstrated considerable sensitivity to income differences.

Income grievances also applied to overtime and other special payments (such as regional allowances) which also influenced migration decisions. As one Fijian doctor phrased it:

> People need to be compensated for their hard work and after hours duty. At present work can be very stressful for those who are trying hard to improve the standards of health care. Why would one put in extra hours of work especially when they are underpaid? The 'good Samaritan' and 'nightingale' days are over.

More than half of the sixty-four Fijian nurses in Suva complained about the low salary and five more about the lack of a shift allowance. As many as twenty-nine felt that they were overworked, particularly for the wages they received. 'Pay and overtime' were routine responses to queries over dissatisfaction, although many recognised that such problems came with the job. Responses were predictable: 'The roster is planned about two or three days in advance so I can't plan ahead'. 'Shift-work is so inconvenient; I can't participate in community things', 'I hate the overtime especially since they only pay us time off in lieu (TOIL)—I work for the money', 'I hate working nights—that's the time to sleep'. SHWs resented long hours of overtime, shift-work, especially double-shifts, working on the early morning 'graveyard' shift or on weekends, especially without adequate income supplementation. Overtime payments (or their absence), that many felt were inadequate to compensate for working challenging and difficult hours, differentiated them from other members of the public service. Older workers were less likely to seek migration and thus more likely to acquiesce to local salary levels, and had managed to stave off excessive overtime. Yet, over time, there had been a slow movement from altruism to professionalism, and from satisfying the needs of the public sector to supporting more private ambitions. Economics mattered.

EMPLOYMENT CONDITIONS

Challenging conditions of employment were the second key explanation for migration. For many doctors earning relatively high incomes in their home countries, this was the main reason. SHWs frequently complained about inadequate support, whether directly through weak management (lack of team-work, poor leadership and motivation, limited autonomy and support, little recognition, poor access to promotion and training opportunities) or through the outcome of poor 'housekeeping' (limited availability of functioning equipment and supplies), extending to a lack of security. Discontent with employment conditions was virtually universal, though the actual practice of health care was almost never a problem. Only in the Marshall Islands did a lone nurse say that the illnesses they were working with could cause them to lose their lives, and that they were not adequately paid for that risk.

After better pay the key reasons for the potential migration of Fijian nurses were 'better work conditions' (62 percent), 'opportunities for further studies and get educated' (24 percent), a better future for family (17 percent), a better career path (17 percent), higher qualifications not recognised (21 percent), stress and frustrations (17 percent), nepotism and favouritism of management (14 percent) and 'victimization and no promotion' (14 percent). Because of these factors, all reflecting variants on the employment context, about a third of nurses left the profession after around five years (Leweniqila, Camaivuna and Dokoni 2000; Lutua 2002). In Vanuatu in early 2008 just two dental chairs were functional but there were no nearby sinks. 'It's no wonder there are only three ni-Vanuatu dentists left, all the rest have left, due to lack of proper facilities and incentives' (*Vanuatu Daily Post*, 12 January 2008). At the small St. Giles psychiatric hospital in Suva, between 1997 and 2000 some twenty-eight registered nurses and orderlies left the hospital, nineteen in search of better pay and improved conditions of work. Fully eighteen of those who left went to New Zealand (where their nursing qualifications would be recognised), three went to Australia and one to Palau. Broadly similar circumstances and responses existed elsewhere.

What constituted poor working conditions were spelled out by many. Overwhelmingly, the main issues of dissatisfaction for nurses centred around physical working conditions and lack of career opportunities; for doctors and ancillary workers access to adequate technology was a critical issue. Facilities were often perceived to be inadequate. Technology broke down and maintenance was problematic, replacements and supplies were not ordered or misplaced. Similar circumstances affected nurses almost everywhere. Most disliked several things about their jobs, well summarized by the diverse concerns of i-Kiribati nurses. Some complained about favouritism within the nursing management regarding promotions and choosing candidates for further training and scholarships. Others complained about being overworked, being required to do overtime and shift-work or being stressed at work: 'you don't get to rest psychologically after working hours'. Two disliked the paperwork; others complained of a shortage of staff, high workload, the occasional unavailability of doctors and the lack of facilities and overcrowding at the hospital (which sometimes ran out of linen and instruments). Two nurses complained about their patients; one said that the job could get repetitive and boring. In Vanuatu, to extend this list even further, complaints included a lack of support staff, and an overall lack of staff and facilities, making it difficult to share one's knowledge and experience, 'no recognition for work done', 'tedious administrative matters' and 'political interference'. While these concerns are valid, no employment context is without some frustrations, blemishes and areas for obvious improvement.

In Fiji the most frequently cited reason, given by more than a third of all doctors who had already migrated, was the poor working conditions in Fiji's public hospitals. But income and working conditions were integrally related. After income, in descending order of significance, were political instability, low salary, inadequate facilities and, finally, the limited scope for postgraduate medical training, all of which contributed to low morale (Naidu 1997: 67). Doctors perceived the primary cause of their emigration to lie in the low calibre of the administrative personnel in the headquarters of the MOH. One observed that 'The Ministry of Health, its Ministers, the Permanent Secretary and most of HQ staff show a level of incompetence which is remarkable even by government standards', and also argued that an emerging social hierarchy where good jobs were going to those with chiefly status, rather than ability or training, was a deterrent to many (quoted in Naidu 1997: 74). Management was never blameless, and management issues were high on the list of complaints, such as the slow and inefficient delivery of requisitions ('too much bureaucracy to approve simple, urgent requests. It's a major source of frustration for doctors'). In Palau, there was 'too much politics in the Ministry of Health' and in the Marshall Islands 'the direction the hospital takes should follow the needs of the people rather than the political leaders'. Those who had trained or worked overseas had seen other administrative structures, which often meant recognising the inefficiencies and unpredictabilities of their own national systems that faced more challenging financial issues. No complex systems are without their failings, especially in the eyes of new entrants with zeal, enthusiasm and new ideas.

Career opportunities were influenced by training. Half of all Fijian nurses were dissatisfied with the lack of training they received, alongside mentoring and the routine acquisition of new knowledge, and situations where there was no adequate system in place to determine who was eligible for training courses. As one nurse explained, 'Nurses are sent on training when near retirement. Younger nurses should go as they have more years to serve'. This feeling that only those approaching retirement benefited from training was echoed by others. Training was not always clearly focused on needs or seen by many of those involved as part of a career structure or part of the continual upgrading of the health system.

> We get a very low standard of health professional here. The quality is so low. There is an inability to understand the long-term objectives of

> training . . . training is an important event but it is not seen as part of any ongoing structure . . . it is an end in itself.

Individualism may be necessary and beneficial, and obtaining senior positions should result from the acquisition of skills and qualifications rather than through kinship connections and nepotism. Another nurse commented,

> [there is a] lack of support and encouragement from the Ministry for nurses who want to pursue further studies. Nurses who go on further studies on leave without pay, or complete degree or diploma training, are taken back on the same salary scale they left on. There is no promotion or increment for studies completed, especially at their own expense. Nurses feel used and it frustrates them. Those who trained overseas tend to leave at some point.

Issues of poor management and administration were cited by many, including discrimination and nurses being posted to departments regardless of training.

> Nurses with specialized training are often taken away to work in other units where they weren't trained. Nurses choose specialized areas and develop interest in specialized areas and train in specialized areas only to find that they are allocated to other units of no relevance to their training, interest and skills.

In small workforces provision of training is difficult where resources are limited and it can be hard (or impossible) to find a replacement. Many SHWs, especially the more skilled, are isolated from professional trends and conscious of missing out on professional development and thus their ability to provide an adequate service or be appropriately skilled to work in a different environment should they later migrate. 'There have never been any opportunities to train since I started in the job . . . I would like to be up to date with the rest of the world'. 'I would like to further my career; there are no challenges here; it's just basic nursing care', 'Few opportunities are given to the young for further training and workshops—we are constantly told "your time will come"', 'Other people go to overseas workshops and training but not me'. Keeping abreast of change and development, especially in the smallest states and more remote areas, is difficult. Where library facilities and Internet access for online journals are particularly limited, as in Kiribati: 'we get deprived of intellectual nourishment'.The chance to work in a better institutional setting and so have better opportunities for promotion and training were major lures.

Management issues are critical for SHWs, rarely if ever motivated by money alone. Empathy and 'good housekeeping' to support skilled workers in challenging situations were often absent. One global review of nurse migration concluded: 'In many countries employers have failed to address long standing deficiencies related to hours of work, salary, continuing education, staffing levels, security, housing and day-care facilities' (Oulton 1998: 126). Difficult and unpleasant conditions have resulted in SHWs being unwilling to work, creating high attrition rates and a 'pseudoshortage' (Chapter 6). Challenging conditions were usually greatest in more remote places, where fewer staff were available and pressures on them usually greater. However, relativities were important since it was usually in the capital cities that nurses complained about difficult working conditions, though conditions in the centre, especially in terms of access to equipment and promotion opportunities, were usually better than in the periphery. Like the patients, SHWs disliked overcrowding, long queues, lack of supplies, inadequate facilities and lack of interest. While in most workplaces it is normal for some expectations to be unmet, especially where workplaces are small, and workers are expected to be flexible, lack of 'good housekeeping' and management was not always supportive of skilled workers in challenging circumstances. Even so, in many contexts, SHWs managed to cope and to stay.

CAREERS, HIERARCHIES, BUREAUCRACIES AND MORALE

The significance of income is linked to the structure of careers and promotion, with many frustrated over future promotion prospects: a standard problem in small workforces with few senior positions. Where it is perceived that promotion is also blocked by being about 'who you know rather than what you know', nepotism, favouritism and longevity in the system rather than ability, frustrations are considerable. Beyond promotion many SHWs sought no more than the respect and support that often seemed lacking, sometimes lost in a generation gap.

In every state many national doctors were aggrieved at the perceived inequality of treatment between local and expatriate doctors, ranging from differences in pay and allowances, the suitability of expatriates' previous experience and the appropriateness of the hiring procedures. As one doctor commented: 'Recruitment of expatriates is often done without proper knowledge of the needs. For example, there are vacant positions that local doctors apply for yet outsiders are being recruited for those positions—often without proper explanation to local doctors why they aren't given those vacant positions'. Another pointed out that: 'Expatriates are treated with favour compared to local doctors yet their performances are not up to standard. If only the same treatment for expatriates was given to local doctors, local doctors will be happy to hang in there for as long as the country needs them'.

Superior status and wages are not necessarily attached to those who have extra experience, and particularly those who have gained extra experience overseas. Indeed, there was resentment over the expectations of those who had returned, in contrast to the perceived greater experience of those who had stayed and 'maintained the system': 'new arrivals start at the same level as those of us who have been here for some time—that is not fair and is why some people are leaving. You can't replace experience'. But returnees saw that differently: 'Those who went overseas are discouraged since they don't get the jobs they should', 'Promised jobs are given to someone else after you come back from overseas training', 'Young ones are pushed to the back—we can't move forwards—old people are ahead'. More generally there were: 'Bad attitudes; people were unsupportive of what I came back with, and my new knowledge, however much I wanted to share what I had got from my new degree, which simply made me want to move away again. I only have one more year of bonding and then I can go back to New Zealand' (thirty-eight-year-old nursing tutor). A familiar concern of returnees was, therefore, that the extra skills and qualifications they had enthusiastically, laboriously and dutifully gained overseas actually counted for very little. Established SHWs had worked for many years, had certain privileges and professed themselves 'too old' to move—yet were resentful of newcomers who sought to make changes that might challenge their particular role.

In small states opportunities for promotion are few because of the limited jobs available, scarce resources and the existing tenancy of those positions that exist. The health profession typically has a 'bottleneck' career structure where there are relatively few senior positions so that promotions are inherently limited. Even in Fiji less than 15 percent of nursing positions are open to promotion (Leckie 2000: 90). In much smaller countries, where there is minimal prospect of promotion in an exceptionally narrow 'career pyramid', accusations of bias, favouritism and nepotism tend to flourish. As a former Niue Minister of Health stated: 'When I was the Minister my uncle was the Director of Health. It was very difficult to be his boss'. (At the time of the study the Acting Director of Health was the only Niuean doctor, who was deputizing for her father, a dentist). While such familial relationships are almost inevitable, in small countries where work in the health sector is often a family tradition, they overlap with professional responsibilities and neutrality is hard to achieve. Concerns over nepotism, whether true or not, are unavoidable in a workplace where several workers are related to each other.

Even in the largest island state a quarter of all Fijian nurses felt that promotions were dealt with unfairly, being based on favouritism not ability. One sixty-year-old staff nurse commented on the:

> lack of transparency regarding promotion. Nurses are assessed every six months yet nurses often do not get promotion or increments for more than ten years. Unless you are in the 'Good Book' or know someone upstairs you are destined to remain a staff nurse for your entire career—no matter how hard you've worked and how well you have performed.

Nepotism was seen by many as a block on personal promotion, while the absence of effective human resource planning was a massive constraint. In Vanuatu it was stated bluntly that 'the government has no overall policy to train these young people . . . there is no structure of forward planning'. Indeed, the Vanuatu Nurses Association has pointed out that:

> Vanuatu does not have in place a proper career path for nursing. Nursing education is therefore NOT linked to any career path, nor is it linked with promotion to the next level. Appointments are made on a 'needs' basis or availability of PSC [Public Service Commission] positions. It is known that in the past and even now, a nurse can be paid at one salary level for a period of up to six to ten years, with no salary upgrading. It has to be said for our nurses in Vanuatu that they are most dedicated to carry on and continue with their duties all these years even with very low salaries and poor work conditions. (Vanuatu 2002)

Doctors had similar experiences; as one observed:

> Posts are for life until you are selected into a vacant high position. Promotions are supposedly on the basis of experience/seniority but not when decisions are made. . .. There's a general sense of frustration—promotions are seen to be made on 'who you are' and 'who you know'. . .. It's very disheartening for junior staff that people are promoted perhaps on the basis of years of service.

Others saw promotions as being more to do with social, even chiefly, status rather than ability or experience (Naidu 1997). In Vanuatu both nurses and doctors complained that they lacked a clear and transparent career structure: 'there is no career structure, no policy direction and no sense of job satisfaction' and another noted:

> There is so much jealousy here . . . everyone wants the good positions, but there is no real understanding or motivation about the structure of the system. I have no respect for those who have gained their jobs for reasons other than merit. It is all about who you know and not what you know.

One ni-Vanuatu nurse actually wanted to be a lawyer in order to help nurses with their claims and support them and others in court cases against management.

In Melanesia nepotism was linked to regional issues. In Vanuatu SHWs were concerned over 'islandism', loyalty to one's own island group and its people above others: the members of an island group—sometimes described as *wantoks* (literally 'one talk/language')—are perceived to work together to support each other. That support may cause frustration for other groups, often smaller social groups that feel and are excluded, and, even on a larger scale, civil unrest. 'Islandism' represents a particular case of positions, promotions and conditions being influenced by ethnicity and kinship rather than merit. In the Pacific, in contrast to extended kin groups and *wantoks,* classes are at best incipient (Gewertz and Errington 1999), while the values that are inherent in class formation—including challenging ethnic and regional boundaries and the hard work, discipline and individualism that enable social change and mobility—must be invoked as the basis of a sometimes elusive modernity underpinning a modern nation (Connell 2007c). Trade unions, however, usually exist in those parts of the bureaucracy that include health workers, and public servants are more likely to strike than most other work groups (see the following). Otherwise, class consciousness is much weaker than ethnic affiliation, traditional hierarchical social structures are powerful and SHWs remain entrenched within kin relationships that significantly influence work cultures and decisions about employment and migration. After the 1987 coups in Fiji 'positive discrimination' in favour of indigenous Fijians had limited promotion and access to training courses for Indo-Fijians, resulting in a greater propensity to migrate. A vicious circle thus emerged with Indo-Fijians being seen as unreliable employees and colleagues and further marginalized. Institutional racism was rarely subtle.

Many SHWs criticized the absence of an evident and transparent career structure, and effectively sought to move to a meritocracy where skills, accomplishments and innovations—their personal social capital—would be rewarded. As one Fijian nurse argued: 'It's hard to make changes here. We try to make changes but other nurses pull you back, because they don't want to change and think you are bigheaded'. Inadequate opportunities for promotion constituted not only an incentive to migration but a constraint to productivity and innovation. Classic 'crab antics' defined relationships in some workplaces. Where any one crab appears on the point of escaping from a container—or as one SHW seeks change and innovation—it is pulled back down by others. Escaping the norm, rising above mediocrity, and even seeking to do so, become impossible, even threatening.

Problems of leadership, or its absence, and the support for junior staff can easily become critical issues in a small workplace with a hierarchical structure: 'Bosses are a big problem; they make life miserable; they don't help; they discourage you more than assist; it's much better when they are not around', 'The matron is inflexible to our ideas and suggestions for change'. 'There is more suppression than encouragement', 'There is too much gossip around—sometimes you simply have to get up and walk away', or just 'nurses have no autonomy'. Quite simply, as an i-Kiribati nurse observed, 'It is difficult to go and complain about anything because this is a small society and everybody knows and there is nowhere else to go'. Some saw this as thwarting efforts at positive change such as shifting from curative to preventative health. Stability in a small workforce with limited turnover discourages change. While some innovations might have failed, and established personnel often had a wealth of knowledge and experience, benefits of training can be lost. Initial enthusiasm wears off and it becomes just another job, much less a vocation, to be tolerated rather than enjoyed. Yet this is universal: in all workplaces some expectations must be unmet.

Ancillary workers particularly tended to be isolated. Most enjoyed the autonomy and the ability to 'be my own boss' but missed the experience of community that existed in other health spheres and had been part of their training. The workplace could be a lonely, isolated and demanding environment, particularly in the smaller states and remote islands where there was often no more than one pharmacist or radiographer, hence individuals had to take on every aspect of the job, sometimes feeling that what they did was not always understood or appreciated. The relative isolation of specialists tended to add to their suspicions that their branch of health care was underfunded or ignored, and that they were overlooked for promotion. As in Palau there are only 'benefits and promotion for the few, and this is not us' and it is 'necessary to find a more supportive environment for psychiatric medicine'. Few liked the paperwork and correspondence they had to do in their positions, quite different from the training that emphasized the practical and curative side of their professional areas. Administration conflicted with practice.

Inadequate numbers of SHWs, not solely (or even primarily) because of migration, inevitably affected the morale of those who remained as they pondered their own future while taking on extra duties and shifts to compensate for the shortages. In the Marshall Islands, the main complaints of nurses concerned the lack of staff and 'frequent absenteeism and tardiness' among the nurses, or of having to do other people's work for them when they did not turn up. Few staff poses particular problems: 'people have no idea when doctors may be resting and call in or phone up at all hours', while those with particular specialisms may effectively be almost always on call. 'I hate the long hours, and the phone calls at night when I want to sleep but it's all part of the job'.

Paradoxically, particularly in smaller islands, boredom sometimes created dissatisfaction, through a low workload. Many health workers, and not merely those with specialized training, had too little work to occupy them. As in some government offices, 'island time' can hang heavily. In the health system this was particularly so at night and resulted in workers dwelling on other frustrations of the workplace, and feeling that they were not usefully contributing, so inhibiting a 'work ethic'. In some more specialized areas there was rarely enough work to enable the maintenance of professional standards: a human version of reverse economies of scale. While this enabled workers to be somewhat flexible over their actual hours at work, flexibility has limits which do not compensate for reduced motivation or the challenges of maintaining standards. 'I like being here [Niue] but I will probably end up going overseas—I want to put into practice what I have learned in Fiji—I need more hands-on experience—we just get bored—there are no emergencies and emergency medicine was exciting'. On the smallest islands this is even truer, as noted by the doctor on one of Tokelau's three coral atolls: 'Four stitches. For me that's a big one. Outside Tokelau doctors don't want cases. But not me, I do. I don't want people to come to harm. But I do wish the nurse would call me at 2 AM and says there's a heart attack' (quoted in Parker 2006: 70). Doctors rarely stay long in Tokelau and the atolls have usually been serviced by temporary expatriate volunteers.

Yet there are always some benefits. For many in more senior positions in government a key attraction of public service employment is overseas travel; many public service workers travel overseas regularly for meetings, conferences and training courses, mostly funded by regional and international organizations. For some, being in the Niue public service constituted being a 'big fish in a small pool'; as one driver who had returned from New Zealand observed: 'Here I am the king of my island; everywhere else someone is bossing you'. Every workplace contained diversity, and most people found some satisfactions.

IN THE REGIONS: 'OUT OF SIGHT AND OUT OF MIND'

Throughout the Pacific, SHWs have been reluctant to move to outlying areas, especially when posted there, because of the relative absence and inferiority of health care facilities, the lack of other services, such as shops and schools (for their families), language and cultural issues, because they may have to work in administrative positions (for which they are not trained) alongside practicing their clinical skills, and because they may be out of sight and out of mind for salary payments, promotion, training, mentoring or conference attendance. Many SHWs in remote areas consequently come from those areas, and accept such disadvantages in favour of a familiar social context and the ability to work with 'one's people'. Thus, though nine out of ten nurses had chosen to work in Vava'u, the second largest island in Tonga, seven went there to be with ill parents, one because her husband was transferred to Vava'u and one had gone back to her original home area. The tenth had married a man from Vava'u. Kinship was a key factor in both attracting nurses to Vava'u and keeping them there. Some had returned to regional areas from overseas, one saying that 'it was important for me to return for my mother. After all, she was the reason why I became a nurse'. Another was satisfied to know that she had 'fulfilled her responsibilities and obligations to her elderly mother and father'. Even so, in Tonga 'no one wants to go to the Niuas'.

In the regions incomes were less likely to be a source of concern, despite complaints about the cost of living (balanced by enforced savings through the lack of availability of certain goods and services), whereas working conditions were rather more problematic. Regional services are not comparable with those in large urban centres. In extreme circumstances, as in Samoa:

> Posting to a district hospital has become a form of exile and sometimes punishment for displeasing a superior, as happened in at least one case which is common knowledge in Apia. (Hoadley 1980: 451)

In such circumstances:

> rural health personnel, especially doctors desiring status and professional stimulation, have sought to rejoin their colleagues at the Apia Hospital . . . Doctors who do not leave the public service display low morale and often turn to social, sporting, commercial or travel activities, leaving their hospitals unattended for varying lengths of time. (Ibid.)

That era is not over, and regional hospitals do not have the status, or the human and physical resources, of those in urban centres.

In Vanuatu social life in the capital city discouraged internal migration, even compared with the next largest town. As one nurse in Port Vila said:

> I liked working at Santo hospital; it is smaller and better managed. We were also better paid at Santo because the management was responsible for our salary increases and overtime payment. I could move back to Santo and my husband could work in the police force but Luganville is not a very interesting place to live. I much prefer the town of Vila. There is much more to do in Vila . . . and much more to spend money on! Santo is very boring.

Rural social life is necessarily constrained. In Samoa, doctors 'miss town', and 'the nightlife' and 'need a fridge full of beer to compensate'. In inland, upland Fiji one nurse noted:

> It's cold and it gets lonely. You're posted to places where we have never been. I found that place to be such a hard place to work in, very challenging. If you have never eaten greens all your life, brother, that is the place where you will eat greens. (Quoted in *Fiji Times*, 7 August 2005)

More frequent complaints about regional life and work came from the most qualified workers: A clear relationship existed between age, experience, specialization and dislike for regions, and having partners who found their own regional challenges. Consequently, 'sometimes I think that I missed out on a lot of opportunities for further studies and promotion because I came back to Vava'u', since 'there's no clear direction for promotion and training', and a degree of centralized favouritism where 'those who make decisions have their own people in line'. In one regional centre the one male nurse was lonely at work, because the female nurses kept to themselves. In the least developed countries—especially Kiribati and Vanuatu—there was even less tolerance of remote postings, and the cultural differences that sometimes accompanied them.

There were compensations for being in the periphery, notably being able to work with one's own family and kin, developing social relationships at work or outside it and, at least in some places, being 'not too busy most of the time'. There was also the converse of what some saw as a remote, uninterested bureaucracy (in Labasa a nurse complained that the bureaucracy took a long time 'to approve things, because it has to go to Suva'), when SHWs were less formally supervised and enjoyed being 'able to plan and implement activities and changes with minimum bureaucracy'. In Vava'u several SHWs enjoyed a 'small, manageable workplace with less bureaucracy' making it 'easier to carry out your work' and 'implement what I want to, to improve the department'. Indeed, the lack of bureaucracy that slowed access to promotion was otherwise often an advantage, as long as it did not translate into the health workers becoming bureaucrats themselves. Even that had its charms: 'I'm the boss, so I'm better able to make decisions and implement them'; jobs could become 'more challenging . . . I am able to make decisions, face problems and take up the challenge'. Ultimately the quieter provincial life held both advantages and disadvantages. Other than for SHWs who came from these regions, and were amidst familiar kin and places, the provinces were nonetheless seen somewhat negatively—sometimes pleasant places to be but stultifying and hard to progress from.

Living in Labasa

The most detailed study of a regional group of SHWs was undertaken in Labasa, and is indicative of some of the diversity of issues concerning living and working in small towns. Labasa, the third largest town in Fiji, has a population of about twenty-five thousand. Though it is the main town on the second island of Vanua Levu, it is much smaller than Suva, the national capital with close to two hundred thousand people, and has experienced some of the impacts of the decline in sugar production.

Of the seventeen nurses in Labasa only six had chosen to live there, ten were transferred by the Ministry and the eleventh followed her husband who had been transferred there. Of the six who did choose to work in Labasa, three did so because their husbands were working there and two to be in their home area (one of whom was looking after an ill mother). When describing what they liked about working in Labasa, eight liked the fact that it was their home area and relatives were nearby. Another, however, said she was 'too close' to her relatives and the land (*vanua*) and had now acquired too many obligations. Other positive factors about Labasa included knowing people: 'because it's a small place, you know everybody here', and the 'slow pace of life'. By contrast, more found working in a small town more challenging simply because they did know everybody. What was positive for some was negative for others. One liked life being 'slower for my children's sake'; conversely, another disliked the 'very slow pace of life' and being 'lonely' since there was little to do after work. The smallness of Labasa had further drawbacks in limited possibilities for further education and the possibility of loneliness; access to kin was only of significance to those nurses who came from the area.

Several nurses enjoyed particular aspects of their work: The 'workload is not too heavy, and 'people respect you for what you do' and it was possible to have a 'good working relationship' with colleagues. None stressed work satisfaction as a reason for enjoying being in Labasa. The most common complaint (from fourteen of the seventeen nurses) was the state of equipment and facilities at the hospital. Medical equipment was 'not up to standard' and both equipment and medicines were in short supply. (The roof of the operating theatre was leaking at the time of the interviews.) Some resented the fact that nurses were expected to clean instruments and linen and another that on-call nurses had to do cleaning on weekends and after hours. A particular—for some unattractive—form of multi-skilling was attached to regional postings.

Doctors and other ancillary SHWs enjoyed Labasa less than the nurses.

> I hate it, because Labasa is boring and the administration is poor, having a colonial- type 'I'm the boss' mentality, which does not encourage progress and does not allow things to move ahead, and yet they talk too much about reform.

The same person also argued that reforms aimed at decentralizing power from Suva had effectively centralized it in one person: 'this has caused frustration not only to myself, but all the staff' because the Director had ignored them. The same doctor was also unhappy that his current job had nothing to do with his area of specialization. And it was impossible 'to keep up with new medical developments and major cases not seen in remote hospitals such as Labasa'. A second doctor said that 'the post is here and it's a promotion', but he was distant from his relatives and there were few educational opportunities for his children. The third liked the fact that the job was 'quiet in terms of workload' and he had got 'used to the quiet life'. However, the job could be more 'satisfying because you know immediately the result', as there was more direct access to patients, hence, you 'know you have made a difference in the life of your community, provided that the machinery is right'. Views about working in Suva were similarly contrasting. One had no interest in going there because 'life is more difficult in Suva', especially for a young family. Another wanted to go to Suva 'because that is where I can be more useful'. The third sought to live in Suva because he had relatives there and it would be better for his children's education. Attitudes to work were as diverse as they were to metropolitan life and employment.

Two-thirds of the Labasa nurses would have liked to work in Suva, because they had relatives there, education for their children was better and further education for themselves and their husbands was possible, enabling development of skills and experiences. Smaller numbers wanted to go to work in a bigger hospital on major cases and get 'exposure' to different medical procedures, and because there were 'lots of places to take your family when you're off work'. Suva was mainly attractive in terms of its superior employment and educational opportunities. A minority (five) of the nurses did not want to work there, because the perceived workload in Suva was too heavy, it was too distant from relatives, more expensive and less safe. What was attractive to the majority was unattractive to others.

Ancillary SHWs such as lab and X-ray technicians were even more likely than doctors to be concerned about their work environment away from Suva. Three of the four in Labasa complained about outdated equipment, one saying 'we always get the rejects from central hospitals' and another 'we are already isolated and then to be dumped with outdated equipment, you feel more remote'. Three complained of the absence of specialists in their areas (such as the absence of a pathologist and of a specialized radiologist for complicated X-ray cases and scans); major cases must be sent to Suva, or specialists brought to Labasa, and 'this means delays'. Limited access to supplies, training and adequate wages completed their negative picture. SHWs in remote postings, even in towns like Labasa that are bigger than some Pacific capitals, are isolated from trends in their profession and in the wider world and are conscious that they may not acquire new skills and training. Isolation, and even boredom, reduce morale and induce migration for many, while a minority feel entirely at home.

In towns smaller than Labasa almost every SHW complained over some aspect of the work environment, with a clear correlation between town size and discontent. Where staff were assigned to regional posts against their will, job dissatisfaction increased despite a sense of duty and the possibility that such regional places could be stepping-stones. Some sense of this comes from the account of the lone nurse on Yadua Island, twenty kilometres off the west coast of Vanua Levu, responsible for a single village of about 160 people:

> I have no problems with my food. The villagers always come around to give some cassava, yams or other crops. I don't know what I would do without them. I always make sure that the supply of drugs lasts and is always in stock in case of emergency. I am on a 24-hour shift here. I treat the patients whenever they come to ask after working hours. I have no choice but to attend to them and sometimes I deliver babies at odd hours of the night. It's a challenging situation and so I see it as a good training ground for me. (Quoted in *Fiji Times*, 14 May 2002: 20)

This nurse was living a hundred kilometres from her home and, like many others in similar remote locations, anticipated that her stay would be temporary—an early phase in a career that would later return her to her home or to a larger centre. While the article in the *Fiji Times* (entitled 'Nurse adjusts to island life') paints a reasonably positive picture of Yadua, others, including the General Secretary of the FNA, are less positive.

> Transport problems are the most stressful at the rural stations because the nurse is often burdened to meet costs of her/his patient when it comes to hiring of transport by sea, river and land. Where there are no roads horse allowance for transportation is sought. The difficulties that nurses face in these remote rural set ups are so unattractive that even nurses who come from nearby villages refuse to serve their own community because of the sacrifices that the nurse has to make in terms of family education as well as her/his own. (Lutua 2002)

Retention of good skilled workers in rural contexts is never easy, and such small islands as Yadua necessarily experience intermittent shortages of SHWs and are always at risk of having uncommitted workers. Labasa is much more favoured.

CHALLENGING THE SYSTEM

Not only are health workers relatively organized and unionized, but they have taken more strike action than other groups. In the Pacific strikes are something of a prerogative of the public service since unions are largely confined to urban areas and few other occupational groups (except miners) are as large or as organized. Nursing strikes have a long history, dating back to pre-independence times in Fiji and Samoa. Not only are nurses perhaps the most unionized group throughout the Pacific but, where women otherwise lack agency and authority, strike action in many countries has had some success. Tongan nurses resigned en masse in 1981, complaining about selection of nurses for overseas training and promotion. As nurses in Tonga subsequently argued:

> It gave nursing a higher profile and struck a blow for women too. Getting those men in government to take notice of us and pay us some respect gave the recognition that we were not to be spoken down to. (Quoted in James 2003: 315)

The ability of a large number of motivated and skilled workers to make themselves heard, though usually working in the same place in an area of national priority, has been considerable. Yet even other, senior SHWs are not always sympathetic. As one observed in Vanuatu:

> People will say that they need more money in recognition of the job that they are doing but nurses know that wages are low in this country. . . . They are working for the good of the country and to help others. When nurses say that they need more pay it is because they are faced with school fees and other expenses. They know what to expect in the government system.

After nurses went on strike in Fiji in 1990 reports of victimization were common, including claims of favouritism with duties, promotion, training and leave being given to those who had not taken strike action (Leckie 2000: 84). In Vanuatu, when 129 nurses went on strike in 1993 (as part of a general public service strike), they all lost their jobs. Many went to New Caledonia to work but most eventually returned. In turn, such government responses have engendered subsequent strike action.

Strikes have raised multiple familiar discontents. Even at the end of the 1950s in Samoa nurses went on strike over inadequate salaries and equipment (Barclay et al. 1998: 35–36). Several times in the 2000s, Fijian nurses have taken strike action, mainly over wages that were cut, as in 2005 and 2007. Persistently underpinning arguments over wages and work conditions, in Fiji and elsewhere, has been recourse to pointing out that migration is one consequence of inadequate conditions. In 2004 the Fiji Minister of Health even responded, stating that there was no solution to migration since 'nurses were marketable and this was a good reflection on the quality of training in Fiji' (*Fiji Sun*, 5 February 2004). In May 2000 the FNA organized a national strike; the government countered with a new pay scale, less than demanded by the FNA, but offered a review of minimum qualifications, fairer rostering, hardship allowances for nurses in remote areas, transport and uniform allowances. Whilst a starting salary, after four years training, of F$10,073 compared favourably with other nursing salaries in the Pacific region, it was perceived as comparing very unfavourably with the starting salaries of doctors in Fiji. 'The nurses became increasingly disillusioned, and also became convinced that they were being taken for granted, possibly because nursing is a predominantly female profession' (Bulicokocoko 2000). The strike ended after three days when the national Permanent Arbitrator ruled in the nurses' favour. Gender issues remain important. As the (male) Secretary of the FNA (96 percent of whose members were women) noted during the 2005 strike:

> I still feel what has been dished out to FNA members and to nurses in Fiji is mostly on gender issues. It's the males flexing their muscles against females and we have seen how females can flex back . . . this is not new for us. (*Sunday Times*, 7 August 2005)

After a similar 1998 strike, Samoan nurses called off strike action in 2000 after the government agreed to a pay increase, tripled the shift allowance and introduced financial benefits for years of service and positive performance appraisals. The existing base salary was T$7,395 (US$2,000) for a nurse with a three-year nursing diploma. As an article in the *Samoa Observer* recorded at the time, their claim:

> was more than demanding a fair wage. It is about respect for one's position and a call for just and fair treatment for the public service in general. And they have a fair argument . . . when your starting salary is between $7–8000 that immediately puts off people in future generations aspiring to this all important position. (Rees 2000)

The Samoan Nurses Association continued to seek a better entry-level salary, relating to their valuable work of nurses and high educational qualifications: 'We still want better recognition of the nurses' contribution to public health and an effort by the government to improve the image of nursing so that young people will choose it as a career'; where there was 'an acute shortage of nurses' 'most of those who have left for training and better opportunities overseas were the young ones' (Anon 2000: 134; So'o 2001: 254).

Doctors' strikes have been fewer than those of nurses. A strike in Samoa in 2005 resulted in a Commission of Inquiry recommending salaries that reflected additional qualifications and length of service, improved staffing levels, reduced working hours, part-time private practice and more overseas doctors (so that local doctors would have time to complete their training). Both the Samoan Medical Association and the government rejected the report, the latter partly on the grounds that doctors were some of the best paid workers in the country (compared with engineers, lawyers and accountants), and the strike continued (*Samoa Observer*, 10 November 2005). Doctors were banned from leaving the country and, after eventual failure to achieve a starting salary increase, at least four doctors moved overseas, three went into private practice and an unknown number resigned. What is true of political systems in small states, that 'the lot of those opposing the group in power is apt to be miserable in the small-scale milieu. There may be no effective refuge, no place to hide, no alternative source of remunerative or prestigious solace' (Baldacchino 1997: 74), is even more true for small-scale health systems within such states. Strikes have only occasionally brought all that the strikers demanded and one recurrent response, as in Vanuatu, Samoa and Fiji, has been increased migration.

THE POWER OF POLITICS

Political factors influence migration in obvious ways (where policies change wages, working conditions etc.) or if political turmoil reduces funding for the health sector or places new demands upon it. Changes in the health sector take place in a wider context where negative balances of payments and trade deficits place huge pressures on countries. In Africa, economic restructuring, imposed from outside the region by international agencies, has led to reductions in the size of the public sector workforce, restrictions on the hiring of new workers and deterioration of working conditions rather than the greater efficiency it was intended to encourage (Connell et al. 2007). In the Pacific externally imposed restructuring has only even come close to this in Vanuatu, with both cuts in the number of SHWs being produced, following reduced national expenditure, and hospitals being unable to absorb even these because of cuts in health expenditure. Similar restructuring of the Cook Islands health system in the mid-1990s meant a loss of career paths and standardization in conditions of employment, a situation that affected staff morale and affected access to services:

> The services are not being used as early as they should be by people to avoid serious illness because the attitude of many staff is hostile and demeaning. The attitude problem has been made worse by many staff being frustrated by poor facilities and low supplies of essential equipment. (SAGRIC International 2000: 18)

Further outcomes were reduced recruitment, increased attrition and migration. Exceptional political events may have exceptional consequences. Coups in Fiji in 1987 and 2000, that were seen as marginalizing that half of the population of Indian origin, resulted in massive migration of Indo-Fijians and especially of doctors, fearful of a long-term future in the country. Many doctors, especially Indo-Fijian doctors, who had left Fiji after the 2000 coup simply cited family security as the primary reason (Oman 2007). While there had been massive emigration from Fiji after the 1987 coups, the 2000 coup effectively reminded many Indo-Fijians that their position was still insecure, migration again followed and the health sector was particularly affected. With the 'nation's health system approaching an abyss', Ministry officials left for the Philippines with the intention of recruiting forty-eight doctors there; Fiji had turned to the Philippines rather than other sources since one impact of the coup was a 12.5 percent pay cut imposed across the whole of the public service. A further impact of the coup, and the resultant emigration, was a decline in health services especially in rural areas, with inadequate diagnoses and a lack of timely treatment (Brown 2000a). An Indo-Fijian doctor who had moved with other relatives to Queensland because of the fear and insecurity that followed the coup, stated:

> It is not good enough to have all the money in the world and at the end of the day be worried you are going to be robbed and bashed. I am leaving with reluctance. I have known the Fiji way of life. I would love to stay in Fiji, because when you are 40 you are well settled. (Quoted in Brown 2000b)

The racial overtones of the coup and the economic crisis it engendered had a particularly destructive effect on the health system, especially amongst doctors, but for nurses, a high proportion of whom were Fijian, the situation was less devastating. Even so, less than four months after the coup, some fifty nurses had resigned, with several being offered jobs either in the private sector or in New Zealand. During the same period, forty-five nurses had emigrated (thirty-two of whom were Indo-Fijians) and had been offered jobs in New Zealand, Marshall Islands, Cook Islands, Palau and Saipan (Northern Marianas). The FNA observed that the remaining nurses were 'overworked and underpaid . . . [and] are refusing to work overtime because they are stressed out. They love their profession and they go out of their way to give their best to their patients' (*Fiji Times*, 9 September 2000). The coup proved a catalyst for a dramatic, and continuing, process of emigration that substantially weakened one of the more effective health care systems in the region. Unexpectedly in subsequent years there was little evidence, at least among the SHWs remaining in Fiji, that ethnicity itself was a factor influencing migration. The 2006 coup in Fiji, without similar racial overtones, drew attention to national socioeconomic problems but did not result in a similar spike in emigration.

RECRUITMENT

In the past decade, as global demand has increased, migration has become increasingly privatised with the growth of recruitment agencies, and their regular use by recipient countries and hospitals. Irrespective of any existing intent to migrate, active recruitment has put growing pressure on, and impressive opportunities in front of, potential migrants. Recruitment agencies smooth the way in attending to bureaucratic issues, satisfying concerns over different countries and cultures, painting a positive picture of unfamiliar destinations and providing induction training. Agencies increase the probability of migration by boosting its potential and providing new possibilities. In the 2000s there has been active recruitment of Fijian nurses for the UAE, a country that few in Fiji would have even heard of until then, and the United Kingdom; in the 1990s there was recruitment to work in several nearby countries, including the Marshall Islands, Nauru, Palau, the Northern Marianas and New Zealand.

> Each year ten nurses are recruited to work at UAE, fetching a $48,000 salary for their families. These nurses transfer a total of $400,000 to the country each year. But the amount transferred was expected to increase as recruiting agents look for more Fiji nurses to work in the Emirates. (*Fiji Times*, 4 June 2002)

Two recruiting agents were ordered out of the country by the Immigration Department, to the consternation of the FNA, whose General Secretary argued that nurses sent back valuable remittances, that the nurses alone should choose what was best for themselves and their families, the government should not 'hold nurses to ransom because it was incapable of handling their concerns' and 'nurses have had enough of the bullying tactics employed by the Health Ministry and are leaving the country like many other technical people because of the lack of better salaries and working conditions'. She did, however, observe that the government was feeling the pinch of the global demand for nurses but 'the right thing to do is address the needs of nursing locally and at the same time negotiate for better deals internationally for exporting services like nursing' (*Fiji Times*, 4 June 2002). Recruitment has continued with a steady flow of nurses to the UAE, and to other parts of the region, and a more limited flow to South Africa, Bermuda and the UK.

Fiji is the only Pacific island state to have experienced recruiting. About twenty nurses a year (out of a national total of about seventeen hundred) are recruited for the Gulf, the Marshall Islands and elsewhere. Most recruited nurses were the more qualified and experienced (*Fiji Sun*, 15 April 2002; Rokoduru 2008) who could get through the necessary language and practical tests, the most demanding being for the more distant countries, such as the UAE, hence only the best nurses were selected.

> Rosemary Waqa experienced a conventional nursing training and early career in Fiji, spending ten years moving between hospitals in Lautoka, Labasa, Suva and elsewhere, before deciding in 1994 that she would work in the Marshall Islands because the income was significantly higher and it would enable her to buy a house. However, after a very short time there serious illness forced her to return. She became an operating theatre nurse in Suva, and completed an Australian (James Cook University) nursing degree programme at the Fiji School of Nursing. A year afterwards in 2006 she was recruited by a New Zealand agency after responding to an advertisement in the *Fiji Times* to work in the UAE. The principal attraction was the salary, alongside free accommodation and transport to work, while Fijian salaries were static and inflation was significant. The aim was to ensure that her two children were properly educated and established. After agency testing and a telephone interview from Dubai (seeking her reasons for wanting to move and her own particular expertise), she went to the UAE, being given a two-week orientation programme at the Sheikh Khalifa Medical City, in preparation for a two-year contract. Other Fijian nurses were working there and at the Towam Hospital in the inland city of Al Ain. (Sheikh Khalifa Medical City describes itself as having a staff of thirty-eight hundred—significantly more than in the whole of Fiji—with its 'senior' staff from western countries and the majority of its staff from Philippines, India and several Middle Eastern countries.) For personal reasons Rosemary only stayed a year in the UAE. During that time, on a salary of about US$26,500 a year, she saved enough money to pay off F$5,000 (US$3,350) on a flat, buy an outboard motor for an uncle, a

> seven-seater van for family transport and about F$2,000 worth of clothes for family members, with some cash remittances for other relatives. She valued the new hospital experiences, such as the new surgeons and techniques, and the wholly computerised technology. She regretted the enormous wastage of goods but enjoyed not having to set out instruments and clean up, that was all done by others, which also enabled a faster turnover of patients. After getting over the culture shock of dress codes and other restrictions, the rigid social structure, demanding patients—where little mistakes of etiquette were not tolerated—and the lack of taro ('you learn to sacrifice in other places') she began to enjoy the different lifestyle, even taking dune buggies into the desert. Back in Suva she was contemplating a new phase of migration to Australia or New Zealand, with the eventual goal of having enough money to establish a backpackers resort in the Yasawa Islands, a significant tourist destination and her childhood home.

At the time that Rosemary was in the UAE, about twenty other nurses from Fiji were also there, some—like Rosemary—Fijian, others Indo-Fijian and Rotuman. Several had returned for a second or third contract, some after finding conditions in Fiji simply too frustrating to return to. A few had been there long enough to be fluent in Arabic, and were gaining new and significant skills, like those of Jane (see Chapter 6). Most were well qualified and experienced even before they had migrated. Even within the region recruitment was highly selective. Fijian nurses recruited for Palau were all Intensive Care Unit (ICU) nurses, recruited on three- to five-year contracts and selected for their skills, and in preference to Filipino nurses, who commanded lower wages. Several nurses who had been first recruited for the Marshall Islands moved on to subsequent contracts in the United States (including Guam and Saipan) as 'cascade migration' became established beyond older colonial ties.

MIGRATION, INERTIA AND UNCERTAINTY

While superior wages and facilities are crucial influences on migration, some have moved overseas for the 'experience', in a rather nebulous sense, but in a process increasingly like that of younger migrants elsewhere in the world who take 'gap years' and working holidays, fuelled by a sense of adventure and a quest for difference and stimulated by the experiences of those who have preceded them. Here as elsewhere the nature of that experience in early adulthood has eventually led to many intended short-term movements, 'for the experience' (whether of superior technology, modern education or simply different lifestyles) turning into much longer and more permanent migration moves, particularly evident in the experiences of Tongan nurses in Australia (Fusitu'a 2000). SHWs are in the relatively fortunate position of being able to gain scholarships or finance such moves through their kin, whether at home or in their intended destinations.

More obviously migration is embedded in strategies for extended household development, where migration is much influenced by the financial needs of family members, whether in the islands or elsewhere. Although economic factors play a key part in explaining migration, as part of what seems a 'standard set' of criteria involving salaries, facilities, career prospects, and also satisfaction and prestige, they do not account for it. The location of close kin and perceptions of family obligations are major influences. Most nurses are women and face particular constraints related to partners' careers and family obligations, which may make remote postings difficult and overseas migration even more difficult. Such social constraints make the link with a career structure more difficult to achieve and increase the sense of frustration. Doctors are twice as likely to migrate as nurses because wage differentials are greater, and because most nurses are women and men are often the primary decision-makers regarding migration (Brown and Connell 2004). However, female Fijian nurses frequently took the decision to migrate autonomously, often leaving their husbands and children behind, mainly for higher wages, but also to escape marriage problems and customary obligations (Rokoduru 2008). Men (most doctors) are more mobile and less sedentary than women (nurses) though many male doctors have migrated to support their wives' careers.

Migration has also been selective by age. In the mid-1990s the mean age of emigrant doctors from Fiji was thirty-four, compared with the mean age of a sample of doctors within Fiji of forty-two. Younger doctors, presumably the more recently skilled, were the most likely to have left. Some 65 percent of all doctors had resigned before completing five years of service and the modal period was just three years. Overseas trained doctors were more likely to have left (Naidu 1997; Tuqa 1999; Oman 2007). Similar situations exist elsewhere, often soon after the bonding period is over. Two-thirds of fifteen Samoan doctors had considered moving abroad at some point in the future (generally to earn some extra money and continue their studies), half were actually intending to migrate (mostly in the next two to three years) and those who had not were either relatively old and/or had trained exclusively in Samoa and had little overseas experience. The existence of a large Samoan population in New Zealand was also a factor, with one doctor in Samoa describing a need for Pacific island doctors to service the needs of the community there.

Both those who wished to stay and those who sought to go—and there was no simple distinction between them—demonstrated uncertainty, ambivalence and a recognition that certain imponderables, notably changing extended family needs, would influence whatever they chose. Thus, a Fijian nurse working in the Cook Islands stated:

> I would love to go next to Australia where I can get extra training and develop my career to become a theatre nurse. My children will really benefit from that and my husband [a chef] could take more cooking

> courses. However, my parents want me to be home in Fiji to look after them so I shall probably have to do that.

Relatively few saw their present location and position as permanent and most at least contemplated some kind of future change. Many had already migrated more than once as part of a cycle of circular migration, in response to different social and economic factors. The repeated mobility of Tevai, a Cook Islands nurse, almost entirely in response to extended family needs, is a classic example of such a migration scenario. Tevai, born on the island of Aitutaki, lived there, in Tahiti and then New Zealand before finishing high school in Australia where she:

> went on to train as a nurse. Tevai had been working in Sydney as a nurse for six months when her father died and she was called back to her family in Aitutaki . . . for the next few years she adopted a dual lifestyle, living alternately in Aitutaki and Australia. In Australia Tevai earned good wages nursing and was able to send part of her wages home to her mother . . . As her mother became ill Tevai found it necessary to spend more and more time in Aitutaki. In 1991 she applied for a full-time nursing job at the hospital in Rarotonga . . . Although she considered the wage to be very poor compared with wages received in Australia, Tevai wanted to live closer to her mother. After her mother's sixtieth birthday the family had a meeting and decided that Tevai had done her share of looking after her mother and that Tevai's sister would come back from Australia to take over. Tevai wants to go back to Australia in a couple of years to earn more money but intends to return to Rarotonga eventually and build a house on the land given to her by her mother. (Hooker and Varcoe 1999: 95)

At virtually every stage in life, therefore, Tevai and her family balanced opportunities for income generation in Australia to provide economic support with the need to be close to family in the Pacific to provide social support. Variants of Tevai's story, and of the transnational corporation of kin, are common: 'I went to Australia for two years and worked in a nursing home but came back when I was needed to look after my uncle's five children' (nurse's aide, Cook Islands). Social obligations underpin these and other migration histories. In complete contrast, where there are no overseas kin, notably for Vanuatu and Kiribati, migration may be almost non-existent. Those few who do migrate internationally usually leave only for training. As one ni-Vanuatu nurse explained, 'we own our land and it is the land that brings us back'. Many SHWs had a sense of loyalty to their country, sought to use their skills to help their people, had a sense of pride and status in their positions and had strong local ties and commitments, all of which provided incentives for staying.

Many islanders have experienced phases of stability, migration and return, sometimes several times, phases that match periods in the life cycle.

Migration tends to be for the young and skilled, and return migration either after bonding or much later (Chapter 6). Despite the transnational corporation of kin, migration is seen as more individualistic, whereas those who stay are said to be committed to community (usually expressed as family, village or church) and nation. Migration and stability can both be seen in a positive and negative sense, with benefits and costs. SHWs remain because the benefits outweigh the costs, but are well aware that this may be a function of a particular time period that relates to the ages of children, the health, age and location of parents and their own particular position (and that of their partners and sometimes children) in the workforce (Connell 2008b). 'I'm stuck here now because of my grandmother—we keep an eye on her—but the rest of my family has gone and we will join them'. Choices over migration hinge on sometimes quite small changes in these contexts, and by the ease or otherwise of migration.

Individuals and households respond differently to similar influences, while the rationale changes over time, perhaps as the distribution of other family members changes or after coups (as in Fiji where incomes and security became more significant than a sense of national duty). Actual migration often has a particular catalyst or tipping point, well illustrated in Fiji:

> It all boils up before a person decides to move . . . to move from one country to another is not a small decision and whoever decides it thinks about it many times by looking at the consequences, and multiplying, dividing, adding, subtracting before they finally make a decision to move, and it's not only one reason that pushes a person to leave the country . . . being born in a country we have pride in our nation and to kill that pride needs a lot of input to suppress that and to decide 'OK I'm not going to serve my country' and move on, move forward . . . It's a multifactorial thing. (Quoted in Oman 2007: 115)

While there are related, inherent cultures of migration the actual moment of migration is never certain.

Ultimately, a wide range of factors influence migration. Income levels and working conditions are pervasive, others more esoteric and individualistic. In Kiribati one nurse feared rising sea levels. Collapse of personal relationships can be a key catalyst. Some seek 'professional growth and development'. Migration can even be an impromptu or passive act, where holidays, education courses or hospital stays overseas, in New Zealand or Hawaii, or periods of leave from the public service eventually become more permanent moves. There are both calculations (of income and human capital) and psychological moments when a tipping point (which might range from cyclones to the death of a particular relative to a particular peak of frustration) becomes the catalyst that turns thoughts and aspirations into actual migration. Migration is rarely a definitive decision; hence, few if any migrate believing that this will be permanent, despite occasional claims of migrants that they have gone for good. Mobility is a constantly repeated and accessible phenomenon, as migrants balance the changing economic and social objectives of themselves and kin: 'once you are a migrant you never know where home is ever again' (Bouras 1986: 12). Only death (and not even taxes) can be certain.

The few studies of migration of Pacific SHWs have actually centred on those who remain in the home islands; hence, there is an obvious bias towards stayers. Yet the many diverse sentiments of disappointment indicate the concerns so many have about their future, that of the health systems and sometimes their country. Concerns are genuine and even heartfelt, and are those of people who retain some desire to provide effective health care, who are frustrated when they cannot do so and who expect to gain personal and household rewards from their jobs, whether moral or material. Throughout the region, numerous SHWs complained over the blocking of professional development, lack of promotion and other problems, and had even taken part in strikes, but while they considered resigning, manifestly they were still there. Fijian doctors who had moved into the private sector acquired a reduced case mix, so that the working environment was less varied than in the public sector, alongside an obsession with payment for service, creating disappointment and discontent that they were not serving a wider public (Oman 2007: 132). As in Fiji the centrality of professional values of service, patient welfare and 'doing good' where it was most needed often overrode what might have seemed their own, and their household's, best interests. Though reasons for migration were never hard to find, a sense of duty remained important, albeit alongside kinship ties and inertia.

It is therefore no real tautology that even within an age and culture of migration most islanders actually prefer island life amongst kin, familiar environments and cultures. Becoming an SHW does not necessarily mean migration. While many did not anticipate that they would migrate in the immediate future, or at all, this was sometimes the appropriate sentiment to utter in view of the close location of their kin. Just as in New Zealand there are public and private views of home, where it is appropriate to publicly state that one is intending to return to Polynesia, but privately do little or nothing about it (Macpherson 1985), so within the Pacific it is appropriate to state that one is not intending to migrate, but actually to be examining the opportunities to do so. Migration is unpredictable, it is both complex and fragile, and ultimately a function of personal preferences that sometimes elude conventional or logical analysis, hence intentions and reality are rarely congruent. Entry into the profession to help the family is as likely to mean stability as migration, and families may deter migration as much as encourage it: 'I cannot leave until my elderly parents have died'. Family commitments are met in various ways. Life crises are crucial catalysts to migration and return migration. Despite cultures of migration, SHWs have been specifically charged with remaining to control extended family land, the ultimate island symbol and substance of security. Both staying at home and going awayprovide opportunities to meet family commitments.

If migration is hedged with uncertainty, intended destinations are not. Throughout the Pacific almost all of those actually planning to leave were going to New Zealand and Australia (due to the ease of transferring qualifications, family members being there and familiarity from previous visits): chain migration dominates despite the rise of recruitment. Outcomes varied, ranging, even for a small group of Tongan nurses in Australia, from 'the complete fulfillment of expectations to the complete shattering of the concept of a better life' (Fusitu'a 2000: 65). Family became even more important in destinations:

> I wanted to give my kids a wider acceptable qualification, give them more options. And I proved it. We did make the right decision. We gave up our jobs though we were probably better off in Tonga. (Quoted in Fusitu'a 2000: 65)

While migrants are part of households and wider communities, the sense of belonging is changing. Younger SHWs, especially doctors who have spent some time away from home, often have a weaker sense of cultural identity, as modernity exudes its undeniable charms. Migration for some even provides a release from cultural demands:

> A whole bulk of people that have moved abroad really have gone because they need breathing space . . . because tradition can really choke you . . . it really shuts you down and pulls you back because in our community . . . your achievements, what you gain in so far as you're obligated to the community you are . . . community property . . . what you gain, what you acquire, what you achieve belongs to the community and people actually just sort of get away from it all, they really go abroad just to have a life of their own. It gets sort of suffocating and chokes you. (Quoted in Oman 2007: 121)

But for most people cultural identity is inescapable and only second generations can shift away from parental roots. One way or another many SHWs have left, and the substantial migration from Pacific island states has had an enormous impact on the region, in terms of the loss of particularly valuable human resources from the health sectors, whether in reduced morale or the very real loss of scarce skills, with implications that this has for other forms of migration (skilled or otherwise), for the countries and for the households of the migrants. These impacts can now be examined in greater detail.

6 The Impact of Health Worker Migration

> Australia, along with New Zealand, has played a vital role over several decades in supporting both undergraduate and graduate medical education in the Pacific, and it is hoped they will continue to do so. Therefore it is of particular concern that to date the medical workforces in Australia and New Zealand have been major beneficiaries of the Fiji specialist programs that they helped to set up. It could even be argued that these programs have served as specialist training sites for these two countries. (Oman et al. 2006: 15)

Migration of SHWs has multiple consequences, from more obvious constraints on the delivery of health services and the economic costs of the loss of locally trained workers to more subtle social, political and cultural impacts. Since migrants move to improve their own livelihoods, and those of their families, they are usually the key beneficiaries of that migration. Recipient countries benefit from having workers who are able to fill gaps and shortages in the health care system. Conversely, sending countries and their populations, especially in remote areas, lose valuable skills unless these are an 'overflow' or are otherwise compensated for. Assessing the impact of all this—even indirectly—is difficult, and numerous anecdotes, at best relating to a particular place at a particular time, tend to take the place of reliable data.

The loss of skilled labour has been of concern for several island states, especially for some of the smallest, who need, but have, few skilled workers. In larger states like Fiji numbers are larger as is migration; of the 8,669 professionals who left Fiji between 1987 and 2001, 2,728 were teachers, 1,774 architects and engineers, 1,410 accountants, 1,137 medical professionals and 1,620 were other professionals (Voigt-Graf 2003). These figures are probably underestimates due to unreliable data sources, and Fiji has also lost airline pilots, accountants, army personnel and sportsmen. The most serious losses of SHWs are of doctors, and in some places much smaller numbers of such workers as pharmacists, radiographers and physiotherapists. The situation is less serious for nurses, simply because every country has many nurses, but nurses are more likely to experience the burden of high levels of emigration.

CONSTRUCTING HEALTH SYSTEMS

While migration has placed stresses on most Pacific health systems it is certainly not the only factor that has limited their effectiveness. Finance is limited and though aid donors have given priority to health, this has not necessarily enabled an adequate 'fiscal space' for the health sector, especially in the least developed and more geographically fragmented countries, such as Vanuatu and Kiribati. Donors long favoured the construction of infrastructure, initially central hospitals, rather than financing the ongoing provision of human resources, technology and supplies. The 'colonial heritage emphasized the monumental hospital, beloved also by politicians because a plaque can be affixed' (Hirshman 1980: 338). In Samoa a central hospital was part of aid that was convenient to give and receive, supported by politicians, planners, doctors and consumers. At some cost to the delivery of rural services, it resulted in an inappropriate urban bias, centralization of health care and a reduction in preventative activities (Hoadley 1980). The technological equipment that comes with large hospitals is more costly and difficult to maintain and service than low technology equipment, especially where maintenance technicians are scarce. Such urban and technological bias has barely diminished over time.

Systemic factors emphasize these structural issues. Reductions in spending on health care systems first became evident in the Pacific in the 1980s and have had a continued and damaging result in sustaining a skilled labour force. The World Bank had concluded by the mid-1990s that the two distinctive features that they identified as the South Pacific health paradigm were 'damaging spending reductions' and 'its vulnerability to worker and/or skill shortages' (World Bank 1994: 19). By the 1980s official vacancy rates were around 10 percent in most countries, and beginning to grow further, with countries having to devise new remedies for labour shortages. Fiji relied on donor support and direct recruitment to compensate for the loss of health workers—with some thirty-six expatriate doctors being made available through the United Nations Volunteers programme in the most critical post-1987 coup period. Samoa and Kiribati kept many doctors in service past retirement age, also turned to expatriates (such as UNVs) who accounted for a third of the public sector (World Bank 1994: 19). Despite such measures shortages were no less evident in the 1990s when migration became more significant.

Limited budgetary support remained critical. In Vanuatu, for example, without significant migration, the number of health workers is inadequate to provide effective health care delivery, and the ratio of SHWs to people is worsening: 'The health system suffers from a lack of qualified staff, especially midwives, doctors and specialists. Basic service delivery is either stagnating or in some cases deteriorating' (ADB 2002b: 2).

Pressure on existing workers raised concern over emigration, or a shift to the private sector, of doctors especially:

> Presently there are some qualified doctors from Vanuatu working overseas—although not for the same reason but due to what one has described as 'poor working conditions'. There is one currently serving in an Australian hospital . . . who left in 1997. In Papua New Guinea there is a report that there are two, while in the Federated States of Micronesia there is one . . . There is also a report that a couple of specialized nurses in the field of anaesthesia and intensive care have left for similar reasons. (*Trading Post*, 24 November 1999: 502)

A female pharmacist later migrated, after being offered only short-term contracts in the public service and being frustrated at receiving a wage lower than her male counterpart. One pharmacist commented: 'She has now passed the Australian standard test, learned to drive and bought herself a car. . . . I cannot see her ever wanting to come back . . . there will be no job satisfaction for her any more in Vanuatu'. Financial crises, and human resource policy, had moved Vanuatu towards a situation like that of the other island states, where emigration is a response to difficult local circumstances. As the ADB observed:

> A number of local doctors have completed training but have left Vanuatu. Recruitment to the profession needs to increase, through the provision of additional scholarships in medicine. Incentives in the public health system should be set at a level sufficient to attract and retain qualified staff . . . The employment structure of MOH needs to be revised, to permit adequate remuneration of qualified doctors and technical staff. (2002c: 243)

Without adequate financial support this never happened, making recruitment, retention training and deployment of effective SHWs particularly difficult. By 2007 the situation was little different:

> At the Vila Central Hospital . . . there are currently some 20 vacancies for nurses out of a total establishment of 70. The active nurses are working under extreme pressure with often only one nurse and a nurse aid on duty on night shifts. Not surprisingly, on average, some 25% of nurses are either on sick leave or are performing at less than optimal capacity due to the severe workload. Due to acute staff shortages at the health centres and dispensaries many nurses are required to undertake higher duties and perform procedures for which they have not been trained. Many of the nurses are past retirement age (55 years old) . . . Nurses on maternity leave are not replaced and the remaining staff members are required to take up their duties . . . With very little supervision and very few opportunities for refresher courses in clinical areas many nurses feel unsupported and not well appreciated. (Rotem 2007)

Even in the absence of any significant migration, lack of resources for training adequate effective health workers has produced a dysfunctional system. While Vanuatu has been more poorly funded than other states (Chapter 2), it illustrates how inadequate funding creates inadequate systems where attrition and migration are outcomes.

Similar problems occur in most parts of the region. In Kiribati:

> The Tungaru Central Hospital is currently being run by a limited number of health staff. The nursing staff are operating at well below the number required, which can be seen by the fact that almost all the retired nurses capable of working have been reemployed. Likewise there have been insufficient doctors due to a variety of causes. One of the main reasons is the poor manpower planning and supply projection by previous administrations, with the result that there are today insufficient clinical doctors with suitable skills, qualifications, experience and motivation to deliver health care at the right place and at the right time. A further main reason for the insufficient number of local doctors has been the very high failure rate (75%) of those studying at the Fiji School of Medicine . . . Very few high school leavers are interested in going into the medical profession. This is not only because of the long and extremely difficult programme of study, but also because of the poor working conditions and limited rewards received after graduation. The premature localisation is another factor . . . resulting in those doctors remaining having to take on an extra load. (Kienene 1993: 254)

While this series of problems explained the shortage, Kienene, himself an i-Kiribati doctor and later the Permanent Secretary in the Ministry, emphasized the emerging role of migration. The government branded the migratory doctors as 'self-centred, reactionary and selfish', a description that was widely accepted, and created later problems for the profession, though their concerns were as much with conditions as with salary (ibid.). Responses to these issues eventually led to the further recruitment of expatriate doctors and somewhat improved overtime wages for doctors.

Problems also occurred in recruiting adequate numbers of nurses. Kiribati requires about forty new nurses a year, but the maximum intake into nursing training is thirty-seven, though this quota had never been met because there have not been enough staff or space at the nursing school. This had flow-on effects to post–basic nursing training, where the official maximum intake was ten students each year but, because of the shortage, only six could be spared each year to undertake post–basic training. Though the shortage of nurses in Kiribati was less severe than that of doctors, some islands were short of nurses, wards had only one nurse on each shift and in others a nurse aide replaced the second nurse. Nurses were often required to work six days a week, rather than their contracted five days. The Deputy Chief Nursing Officer observed that in 2002 in the private ward they needed thirty nurses and had nine or ten, in paediatrics they needed seventeen and had thirteen and in the operating room they needed seventeen and had ten. Consequently 'too many nurses have not taken their leave since 1999' (Easthope 2002). A shortage of ancillary SHWs and dentists led to the National Health Plan observing that: 'The X-ray unit is run mostly by unqualified staff', the X-rays were of poor quality, the machines were often out of order because there were few engineers to repair and maintain them and there was no technical assistant for the radiologist (Government of Kiribati 1999: 61). As in other states, where such frankness in national plans was lacking, the situation in the more specialized areas has been of particular concern.

An adequate supply of trainees is a much wider problem. It was estimated in the 1990s that the Majuro Hospital would require 145 nurses by 2000 but in early 2002 it had just seventy-seven: a 'critical problem' (*Marshall Islands Journal*, 10 May 2002). A leading article in the national newspaper stated:

> The ongoing shortage of nurses at Majuro Hospital presents two difficulties: one is the immediate and ongoing pressure that it puts on the ability of staff to maintain a basic level of service to patients; the other is the problem that not enough Marshallese are going into the nursing profession, forcing the hospital to rely heavily on expatriate nurses. The reality of this situation is that often nurses are left to work double shifts (16 hours or more) for lack of staff. (*Marshall Islands Journal*, 3 May 2002)

The shortage of Marshallese nurses was related to low educational achievements in high school (that made it difficult for high school leavers to succeed in tertiary level courses), low salaries compared with other professions and the amount of work that existing nurses were seen to be doing. Although recruitment of doctors is rarely difficult in most countries, because of higher salaries and greater prestige, in Micronesia it faced graver problems than for nurses, for the same reasons. Dentistry faced similar problems; as potentially the first indigenous Marshall Islands dentist observed, 'I hope I can set an example and make kids more interested in going to school [tertiary education]' (*Marshall Islands Journal*, 1 February 2002). Shortages of local SHWs were almost predestined by the education system.

Even relatively strong budgetary support may be inadequate. In Tonga, although the national health budget is second only to that of education,

> These funds are grossly inadequate to enable hospitals to provide patients with even the most basic standards. For example, there have been no funds for hospital linen for four years, and at times the hospital does not have money to buy basic cleaning materials or stationery to keep patient records. (Harkness 2001: 37)

In the Marshall Islands and FSM, as elsewhere, most expenditure is on salaries (and referrals) with little allocated to maintain facilities, buy equipment and supplies and train staff, hence hospitals and dispensaries:

> constantly experience supply, equipment and drug shortages. In some areas such as Chuuk facilities have been left abandoned due to the lack of funds to provide equipment and staff. Even when equipment is available the lack of maintenance and supplies needed to run these sophisticated machines are often neglected. Overall health services on FSM and RMI have remained outdated, are in dire need of repair, and experience frequent power shortages. (Tokuda, Cernada and Kurahara 2001: 208)

Similar epitaphs might be written for some other parts of the Pacific, especially beyond capital cities.

Conversely, as financial crises have affected the public sector so the private sector has grown, accompanied by some migration of SHWs from public to private. Costs of consultation at the MedCen private hospital in Apia were approximately ten times those of the public sector (though, in a new hospital, facilities were considerably superior); commensurate wages meant that the hospital attracted some of the better Samoan doctors. Nurses too moved from the public to the private sector, both to MedCen and to a private school for American students: 'Nurses from the National Hospital have been attracted to the school because of the good salaries it offers. This became a concern for the health authorities who kicked up a lot of fuss over the issue' (Fatupaito 1997: 21). Pharmacists have been particularly prone to shift between sectors. Fifteen of twenty-five pharmacy graduates from FScM quickly moved into the private sector because of non-recognition of qualifications in the public sector and inadequate career progression grades; three others had migrated (Bailey, Khaiyum and Prasad 2006). A similar pattern of movement from public to private sectors is evident in other sectors, such as legal practice, education and IT, alongside a shift into regional institutions and small business, none of which provide the basic training costs (Liki 1994: 66–72, 143), though there may be national benefits.

Just as there are limited resources to develop adequate health care systems, so potential patients have limited resources to pay for services. Even minimal payments may discourage attendance until illnesses are serious. In Port Vila, for example, patients are reluctant to visit clinics such as that of Wan Smolbag because of the 200 vatu (US$1.75) payment or the Vila Central Hospital because of the 500 vatu payment. Transport costs (about 1,000 vatu return from eighty kilometres away, when the roads are in good repair) further limit visits from rural areas, and the costs of servicing them. In American Samoa patients from the second island group, Manu'a, are often unable to afford the US$140 round trip to the main island to visit the lone hospital. Despite a monthly visit from a doctor, costly medical evacuations are common or treatment is simply absent (*The Samoa News*, 2 November 2005). Remote regions are consistently disadvantaged. Systemic problems of low budgets, limited recurrent funding (for salaries, equipment and supplies), weak education and management systems deliver health services that are less than adequate.

TOWARDS CRISES?

While losses of SHWs were evident in the 1970s, the first impacts were probably only documented after the 1987 coups in Fiji that provoked significant emigration. The health service consequently deteriorated, because of the loss of workers and the economic decline that reduced health budgets. Anecdotal evidence recorded poorer service delivery, excessive overtime and poorly maintained facilities.By the mid-1990s, a senior official of the Fiji Medical Association stated that a crisis looms in 'our hospitals and the Government does not seem to want to address it' and added that 'the shortage of adequately skilled and experienced doctors was affecting the quality of care' (*Fiji Times*, 30 September 1995). Since migration was dominated by Indo-Fijian doctors, a secondary consequence of the coup was that senior vacancies were filled by underqualified applicants on the basis of ethnicity rather than ability (Naidu 1997). The resignation and migration of doctors led to inefficiency, low productivity, poor morale and greater frustration, a vicious circle that was only stimulating more migration, while the absence of key individuals had a 'domino effect' through the under-utilization of particular units (wards, labs etc.). Regional areas experienced such crises more forcefully. The Prime Minister, Sitiveni Rabuka, maintained that:

> The emigration of doctors is a drain on Fiji's professional and human resource. Some say the reason they left the country is political. This is an easy excuse that is really a rationalisation of the real reasons for emigration, and that is the wider opportunities for a more comfortable life overseas. I believe doctors who were born here should show more dedication to Fiji and make their contribution to their people, rather than going off to sell their services to richer people in those countries. (*Fiji Times*, 13 May 1996)

Such appeals to altruism had no effect in a context where positive changes to the health system, or to the wider national economic context, were lacking, and construed as an unwillingness to deal with more complex social and political issues.

The loss of nurses was never as critical in Fiji; proportionately fewer nurses left because more nurses were Fijian. By contrast, nurses left more steadily; while less concerned over the obvious politics of the coups they were frustrated with its consequences—the increasingly 'normal' problems of 'unsatisfactory salary structures, low salaries completely incompatible with acquired scarce skills, poor career paths and promotional prospects, unacceptable allowances, poor working conditions' (Bulicokocoko 2000). Grievances were more likely to be articulated through strike action than migration (Chapter 5), partly because many nurses were married and saw migration as an impossible option. Migration nonetheless increased and, ironically, as elsewhere, problems experienced by nurses were partly a function of that migration, reaching 'crisis proportions' when 'the workload of the nurses increased dramatically due to the large number of skilled nurses migrating for greener pastures abroad [hence] those who remain have therefore been required to work additional hours with added responsibilities in order to try and cope with all nursing care services. Nurses became overworked on forced overtime and continued to be under paid with poor transport' (Bulicokocoko 2000). Such issues escaped formal documentation.

The sharp jolts to the Fijian health service that followed post-migration emigration were, with the exception of the Solomon Islands, not paralleled elsewhere. Steady attrition and migration thus produced less focus on the impacts. However, in Samoa, 'Whilst there have been significant numbers of Samoan doctors trained since independence, losses of doctors to other countries in the region and to rim countries continue to be a major problem' (World Bank 1994: 315). Moreover, migration meant that by 1991 most Samoan doctors practicing in the public system were either above the retirement age of sixty (fifteen out of thirty-four), having been brought back from retirement to cope with the shortage, or new graduates (eight of the thirty-four being aged less than thirty-five), so that more than a third of all public sector doctors were United Nations Volunteers (World Bank 1994: 315). Similar problems affected nursing. In 2000 the Samoa Nurses Association pointed out that there was a very significant nursing shortage (with one hundred vacancies out of four hundred staff), hence family members had to attend to sick relatives in hospital, nurses consistently had to work overtime, the demands being such that many had moved overseas or gone to work in private businesses. A survey conducted in 1997 by the Division of Nursing showed that most of those who had emigrated were younger nurses, for training and better opportunities: 'the bottom line is money. Just like doctors, according to an NUS [National University of Samoa] official' (*Samoa Observer*, 7 May 2000). In Kiribati a lack of doctors posed problems. Only one doctor covered the psychiatric ward, paediatrics and emergency, and Kiribati had only four specialists (medicine, surgery, paediatrics and obstetrics and gynaecology). Patients often had to be referred to Fiji or New Zealand, 'sometimes without a clear diagnosis' and at a significant cost to the MOH. A lone doctor worked in the very busy major urban centre of Betio, covering everything from outpatients to emergencies.

In Tonga, where earlier migration of nurses had apparently presented no problems, by the late 1990s the situation had changed. As many as twenty-five nurses are said to have emigrated from Tonga in the one year 1998–1999 (Rotem and Bailey 1999: 18), and Tonga's health workforce situation was perceived with gravity:

> Issues relating to staff morale, staff productivity and staff attrition rates are clearly recognized as problematic areas for the ministry. Anecdotal evidence suggests that staff morale has been very low. The reasons are felt to be multifactorial, however, issues relating to human resource management have been indicated as significant. Poor punctuality and high absence rates from some employees are a source of considerable frustration and irritation to many staff. . . . It is felt that there is a disparity of staff deployment across the system . . . there are definite areas with staff shortages and a lack of adequately trained staff . . .. Another significant area of concern is the high level of attrition. This has long been an issue with respect to medical staff, but is also becoming a major problem for nursing staff and other allied health and technical workers. Low financial remuneration is cited as one of the key reasons . . . but there are other reasons relating to workforce management and communication. Lack of any career development may also be a contributing factor . . . The maintenance of an appropriate skill base within the health system is one of the greatest challenges facing the Ministry. (Tonga. Ministry of Health 2000: 44)

The workforce situation has not subsequently improved. What was true in Tonga was generally true elsewhere. Workforces were declining, and aging, relative to population growth, as migration accentuated budget and management problems. It was implicit, if rarely explicit, that services were being delivered less effectively.

HEALTH CARE PROVISION

Migration affects both the quality and quantity of health care. Lack of workers disrupts and reduces health services. Logic and anecdotal data suggest that there are strong links between migration and the reduced performance of health care systems but actual correlations are impossible to make. Numerous articles make such a correlation but without obvious evidence (e.g. James 2003: 318; Pak and Tukuitonga 2006). In some countries, notably Fiji, daily newspapers have long been replete with headlines, cartoons and photographs of long lines at health centres, accounts of the closure of remote health centres, references to overcrowded waiting rooms, unavailable health personnel, delays in attending emergency cases, lengthy waits and cursory examination and treatment, a situation that causes inequitable access to health care. Such anecdotal information, newspaper stories and photographs usually reflected worst-case scenarios, but responded to perceptions of malaise that were poorly documented formally where changes might be subtle but steady.

MORALE AND MORTALITY

Migration of SHWs contributes to loss of morale (albeit also immeasurable) among those who have stayed, and even fatigue, stress and overwork, and the assumption that circumstances can only worsen if more people go. In turn, this accentuates the migration system. Initial migration makes it more difficult for that system to function effectively, and may herald a downward spiral of its capacity and a corresponding upward spiral of migration. (This is particularly so where migrants formally go 'on leave'—the phenomenon of 'ghost workers'—and cannot easily be replaced until it is clear that they are not returning.) Older and more experienced nurses tend to retire, while younger more recently trained SHWs tend to migrate, hence numbers alone do not reflect the workforce situation. One way or another, the best and brightest are more likely to leave.

Overwork has taken a toll. Staff shortages lead to excessively long hours, fatigue (and possibly wrong diagnoses and decisions) even manifest in physical symptoms:

> There were times when I was really stressed out . . . where it really showed up physically and I started to develop . . . infections, abscesses . . . so that it really showed how much I was stressed out. (Quoted in Oman 2007: 92)

There are at least implications of declining quality of care, while stress led to unmanageable workloads, and more resignations followed by even worse workloads. In 2004 eight Fijian nurses, all aged between forty and fifty, died—a situation attributed by the FNA, at least in part, to the burdens of additional work. The increased overtime work and restrictions on leave thrust upon workers, as in Palau, were not only causing 'fatigue and a general decline in morale' but overtime payments resulted in an added US$300,000 to the general budget (Miho 2007). Social and economic costs were combined.

Activities are foregone or cannot be discharged effectively. In Fiji the emigration of SHWs, alongside internal migration of islanders in response to new economic circumstances, meant that some new clinics received no new staff and overall fewer SHWs were available to vaccinate children. In the early part of this century the vaccination coverage rate fell from 95 percent to below 80 percent, and in 2006 Fiji reported many new cases of measles, from which it had been free since 1998. To return the vaccination rate to normal took a massive mobilization of SHWs and some other work was put on hold for three months (Ken 2008). A shortage of anæsthetists in Fiji has meant the cancellation of operations (Oman 2007: 113). The impact of migration was greatest in areas such as paediatrics where, while migration similarly worsened workloads, the impact on mortality was less obvious, despite decisions having to be made about whether to close the outpatients department or the ICU at the main Suva hospital (Oman 2007:

114). Migration also both directly reduced the number of qualified supervisors and tutors and indirectly reduced the amount and quality of guidance and mentoring.

Inability to deliver services had one further crucial outcome, at least in Fiji. Some doctors resigned who felt they could no longer cope with the combination of a massive workload, and the perceived consequence of an unacceptable degree of patient mortality. As a senior Fijian consultant said: 'I think they felt there were a lot of deaths and morbidity that could have been prevented if they were just more vigilant . . . but there are some things that will break you' (quoted in Oman 2007: 110). Staff and patients are joint victims of inadequate human resources.

The shortage of doctors, especially specialists, has meant that some procedures cannot be undertaken in island states, hence referrals have been necessary. There is no data enabling any correlation of referrals with the loss of SHWs, and the extent of referrals is more likely to be related to budgetary policy. Where they are at the expense of the state the cost is considerable. Even where they are not, as is sometimes the case, household resources are nevertheless transferred overseas from the island states. Overseas referrals continue to take up large proportions of the budget in several states, especially northern Micronesia. In most parts of the region they make up as much as 20 percent of budgets, despite some reorientation to India and the Philippines and the role of visiting health teams (Chapter 2). Referrals within states can also be expensive. In 2000 in Samoa, where international referrals absorbed as much as 20 percent of the health budget, various procedures could not be undertaken on the second island of Savai'i, hence, there were also costly transfers from that island (with many parallels in the region). For most small states this would have occurred in any case, but it represents a substantial loss of scarce resources that would diminish with local access to adequate care.

REGIONAL DECLINE

In centralized systems the burden of migration (and inadequate management, finance and governance) has fallen most heavily on more remote areas where disease burdens are usually greater, and services already least adequate. As in Samoa, provision of services in remote areas is particularly inadequate, and SHWs in remote areas had limited contact with the centre and felt excluded from the system:

> Staff development . . . is not happening and needs to be addressed . . . Most of the nurses work alone and have no access to medical personnel so they really need to upgrade their skills and knowledge. A decent salary should be a good motivation for people to do the training and then stay in the remote areas. Accommodation for the nurses should

> be upgraded to enhance her [sic] job satisfaction. This should include providing all necessities. (Kerslake 1993: 92–96)

Shortages of SHWs were most evident in the regions, with two outcomes: heavy workloads and lack of mobility. In Vava'u there was only one nurse per ward per shift. A shortage of staff in Labasa meant that sometimes patients got aggressive. That shortage meant that there was little incentive to move regional SHWs to the centre, and their voices were not always heard. One regional ni-Vanuatu nurse, who had upgraded to a more senior position, noted:

> Ever since we completed this programme I have had no salary increase, so there is no motivation to improve one's education. In the work setting the support is not there. Transport is poor and I work here by myself and sometimes for months you don't see anyone. We are poorly supervised and poorly supplied with equipment. (Quoted in Kerslake 1993: 72)

Monitoring and mentoring were rare. In 2000 the second national Samoan hospital, on the island of Savai'i, was without obstetrics specialization or a surgeon. The resident doctor was a young man whose family had remained in the capital. He was described by a senior public servant in the Department of Health as 'serving about two hundred people a day, an enormous burden for a young graduate. Since he is always on call he sees his family about once a month. While remote folk believe their work will be recognised it is not. They are effectively out of sight and out of mind'. The health needs of almost a third of the national population were relatively poorly served, while such people rarely stay long (either there or within the country). Lack of contact and moral support emphasize that rural areas fare worse than the centre.

Technology and supplies were less adequate (especially where stock control and ordering systems were absent), and SHWs complained over neglect—to the facilities and to themselves and their career prospects (Chapter 5). As one doctor in Aitutaki, Cook Islands, noted:

> We need two doctors here; there is lots of work and we need public health too. I should be visiting patients but I can't leave the hospital because there is no time. I have to refer surgery and maternity cases to Rarotonga because we do not have adequate facilities and I think I am beginning to lose these skills now.

Inadequate access to technology and medicines, poor facilities (with the diabetic clinic 'tucked away in the laundry room' and a lack of transport for community health visits) all frustrated job performance. Similar problems reflect economies of scale, real difficulties in meeting the recurrent needs of remote places and the task of organizing adequate health care in the face of staff shortages and the regular mobility of personnel.

Staff shortages have affected hospitals even in relatively large centres. Waiting times have become longer, typified by a patient at Lautoka hospital (the second largest in Fiji) stating: 'I have been waiting for four hours and have not yet been seen by a nurse or a doctor' (quoted in Ken 2008: 43). Others stop waiting or simply do not attend. In Labasa in 2002:

> More than 60 patients were told by Labasa hospital staff to see a private practitioner because they could only attend to emergency cases yesterday. There was only one doctor on duty and more than fifty people sitting and lying on the benches waiting for the doctor. The Director of Hospital Services said two doctors were being sent to relieve the problem. He also said that five doctors from India would fly to Labasa to ease the problems faced by staff and patients. (*Fiji Times*, 28 March 2002)

However, by the middle of the year:

> Long queues continue to be a sight at Labasa Hospital with the doctor shortage a major problem. A number of patients said they spent long hours waiting before they could see a doctor at the Outpatients department and at special clinics at the hospital. The frustrated patients said a number of times they had to go home without being attended to by doctors. (*Daily Post*, 3 July 2002)

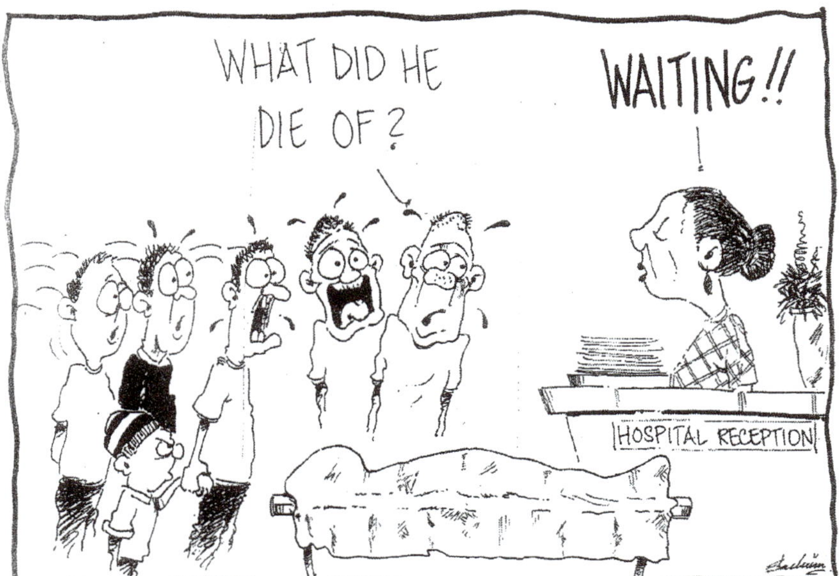

Figure 6.1 The long goodbye.
Credit: *Fiji Times*, 24 July 2005

Smaller hospitals and health centres are even more difficult to staff. Rotuma, the most isolated island in the country, had one doctor and supplies could be delayed for a month (*Fiji Sun*, 17 May 2002). Nurses have less time to make visits and work with communities, hence preventative health care, and the poor receive less attention.

One outcome of worsening regional and rural services is that in Fiji, PNG and probably elsewhere, members of rural communities have increasingly chosen or had to bypass their officially designated clinics to ensure more adequate treatment at regional centres, and so 'fight all odds to attend [regional] hospital outpatient departments for medical consultations, even for their basic or minor health care problems' (Tuqa 1999: 7). In a sense rural problems became urban problems, at some economic cost to patients (both directly—transport and even accommodation—and in terms of opportunity costs), resulting in the under-utilization of rural health centres and congestion and inefficiency in the hospitals (as at Labasa). This further emphasizes that the more remote and worst facilities are for the very poor (and under-utilization suggests they need no new resources), while the prestige of the central hospital, and its staff, has risen at the expense of district hospitals. Similar effects occur where there is any relatively prestigious central hospital that may create its own demand (Hoadley 1980), with an ensuing vicious cycle of limited attention given to regional facilities where demand is falling. The ramifications are evident in the manner in which life expectancies have failed to increase and may be declining in peripheries. (In PNG, Vanuatu and Solomon Islands there has been an actual decline in the number of rural health facilities and in the resources of those that are operational, with negative outcomes.) As migration has taken more SHWs from rural and regional areas and servicing them becomes more difficult—or simply ignored—so a downward spiral of reduced morale and further migration is initiated, and equity is less well served.

ECONOMICS

The most basic impact of the migration of health workers is financial. Training is lengthy, and often overseas, scholarships and costs are high (even relative to most other skilled workers); hence, when SHWs migrate (or resign or even take early retirement) it is a costly burden for poor states. At the rate of resignation that was operating in Fiji in 1999, when twenty-three doctors had resigned, the annual cost to the government was estimated to be around F$13,674,000 (US$7,000,000) in additional training costs at the FScM alone. Meanwhile, hiring of expatriate doctors cost an additional F$2,657,700 (US$1,400,000) per year, over and above what it would have cost to employ the same number of local graduates (see the following). However, actually calculating that financial burden for doctors alone is exceptionally complicated (Connell 2008c: 18–19), since heroic assumptions must be made about the costs of tertiary training (and earlier education), let alone much more subtle costs arising from health care foregone, repeated staff changes, the duration of future employment and the value of replacements.

One estimate of the total cost of international migration for Fiji is that Fiji was losing around F$45 million (US$30 million) a year in the late 1990s (Mohanty and Naidu 2005: 158–160), with perhaps about a quarter of that accruing to SHWs. However, the methodology is not described while indirect costs (such as work foregone through ill-health by people who would otherwise have had access to health care) are excluded. Furthermore, the value of return migration is excluded, though it is slight, while remittances are considerable. No estimates have been made for other parts of the region. Crude attempts to balance the costs stemming from migration suggest substantial losses in training costs, and significant losses in activities foregone, despite replacement. While remittances, certainly from nurses, are considerable and sustained over time (see the following), so that their overall volume is probably greater than education and training costs, they largely benefit the private sector (Connell and Brown 2004). Nonetheless, despite the considerable social costs being ultimately immeasurable, there may currently be a net economic inflow into the Pacific source countries. Yet, at the same time, the migration of SHWs remains a perverse flow of scarce human resources from relatively poor countries to relatively rich ones, representing a massive economic gain—even a subsidy—to metropolitan states, through their own very substantial savings in education and training costs.

REPLACEMENTS

In every Pacific state the lack of SHWs has been compensated for by replacement with migrant SHWs from elsewhere. Part of this circulation is within the Pacific, as Solomon Islands doctors have gone to the Cook Islands, Fijian nurses to Marshall Islands and Palau, and ni-Vanuatu nurses to New Caledonia and the Cook Islands. A Samoan doctor works in Niue. Filipinos were there previously. Samoa had eight Indian and four Chinese doctors in 2007. Marshall Islands has recruited nurses from the Philippines, Fiji, Solomon Islands, Tuvalu and Kiribati. An i-Kiribati nurse is in the Cook Islands. American Samoa, though with enough doctors, recruits all specialist positions—such as pathologists and surgeons—and also nurses—from elsewhere in the Pacific, particularly Samoa and Fiji. However, it has generally been easier and cheaper for Pacific states to remedy labour shortages by recruiting from Asia and even beyond. Consequently, there are Taiwanese doctors in Solomon Islands, Japanese in the Northern Marianas, South Koreans in Palau, Filipinos and Pakistanis in Fiji, Bulgarians and Russians in Vanuatu and the Cook Islands and Burmese in the Cook Islands: all part of cascade migration. By 2003 a third of all doctors in Fiji were from overseas, including the Philippines, Nigeria, India and China. In the same year eleven of Palau's twenty-six doctors were from overseas, including three from the United States and one each from Burma, Fiji, Korea, PNG, the Philippines, Marshall Islands, Solomon Islands and Vanuatu. Fourteen of Palau's sixty nurses were from Fiji, even though the Northern Marianas were then paying higher wages to Filipino nurses and 'we are missing out'. Others from New Zealand, Australia, Canada, Germany, Norway and elsewhere are employed, usually under particular aid and volunteer programmes.

Cuba particularly has extended its global scheme, which by 2005 had reached sixty-eight countries mainly in Africa, Latin America and the Caribbean (Ospina 2006), into the Pacific. Nauru was the first state to take Cubans, but the contracts of eleven Cuban doctors were terminated early, since they were not seen as 'team players' and their English was poor. The Solomon Islands, with 196 vacant positions, requested forty Cuban doctors in 2007 and were offered ten, alongside fifty medical scholarships for students to study in Cuba. Cuban doctors were seen to be cheaper and therefore more cost-effective than other possible international recruits, and with knowledge of tropical diseases such as malaria (Wasuka 2007). Kiribati recruited ten Cuban doctors in 2006 and PNG some twenty in 2007, rejecting a request by the Australian government to abandon the plan because it would 'destabilise security in the Pacific' (*Sydney Morning Herald*, 11 July 2007), and at the start of 2008 Vanuatu was offered five doctors (and ten scholarships). The Cuban doctors in Kiribati worked in the central hospital, but in Vanuatu, PNG and Solomon Islands they were all intended to work in regional areas.

Overseas recruitment has been difficult given the salaries that Pacific states are able to pay, and pressure from local doctors that these salaries be similar to their own (Chapter 5). When a group of Bangladeshi doctors were recruited for Fiji in 2005, the Fiji Medical Association demanded that the government pay them the same salary as local doctors, since 'they should have equal pay if they have the same qualifications as overseas doctors. If not we will lose them to the private sector and worse still we might lose them overseas' (*Fiji Times*, 24 November 2005). The salaries and conditions (such as access to housing) of expatriates may reduce the morale of similarly qualified local workers, who perceive themselves as more able to deal with local circumstances. A year later recruitment of doctors from the Philippines and Bangladesh emphasized other problems. Two trips to both countries were made to recruit forty-seven doctors (a vacancy rate of 16 percent) but had achieved limited success 'given the fact that Fiji was competing with countries with more financial resources in attracting doctors from the same human resources pool' (*Fiji Times*, 14 June 2006). Irrespective of the value of expatriate doctors, and other health professionals, there is always considerable expense (in time and money) attached to their recruitment, including sometimes long delays, the difficulty of finding the right recruit, the cost of recruitment and so on. This is fraught with problems for small states such as Kiribati: 'Finding expatriates with the necessary skills and aptitudes can be difficult. Donors that provide fully funded experts sometimes only provide one candidate for each post, thus restricting the choice of the recipient' (Bakeea 1991: 258). This puts considerable pressure on bureaucracies who are sometimes poorly equipped to cope. The indirect costs of migration can be considerable.

While doctors recruited in Asia are paid salaries broadly comparable to local doctors, those recruited in Australia are paid substantially larger salaries. At the start of 2008 an Australian surgeon in Vanuatu on a salary of A$150,000 (plus benefits) would earn about five times the salary of the best paid local doctors. While, as in the case of most Australians, the cost of hiring overseas professionals is borne by overseas aid funds, the direct and indirect costs of hiring overseas SHWs can be considerable. In Solomon Islands in 2001 hiring nine foreign doctors took up 22 percent of the salary budget for doctors, while the seventy-three national doctors absorbed the remaining 78 percent. In 2003 in Tuvalu two expatriates, specialists in anæsthesia and surgery, were each paid A$90,000 while local doctors earned A$12,000. Moreover, opportunity costs are attached to even the donor funds that support the expatriates, hence Kiribati, at the start of the 1990s, had to rely on a doctor workforce a quarter smaller than that in place a decade earlier, because its salary budget was exhausted.

Most expatriate SHWs have moved for a combination of financial reasons, especially for nurses within the region, and the experience. Altruism was more true for doctors from developed countries. Fijian nurses in Palau, all of whom were ethnic Fijian women, had come in some part for the much superior wages but they usually also expressed other reasons: 'I actually became a nurse so that I could travel', 'the travel experience', 'better education opportunities'. Many had become nurses as much for the financial and other rewards as out of any degree of altruism. Migrant doctors were in Kiribati for three reasons: the experience, to help people worse off than themselves and to be with their families. Altruism and enthusiasm for new challenges were not unusual despite the basically economic rationale for migration. Of eight doctors who had come to work in Fiji (three from Burma, with the remaining five hailing from such diverse locations as Hungary, Pakistan, the Philippines and Nigeria), one had come to escape the 1988 coup in Burma, three had been posted by the UN and four had applied for jobs simply as a change, a chance to earn better wages or to reunite with family. None had been to Fiji previously and most typically had little knowledge of it before arriving. One European had been divorced, sought a change of scene, found Fiji in a tourist guide and wrote offering his services. While some migrants eventually stay on, a long-term commitment to the Pacific is unusual. In Palau, the few who had considered the possibility of staying beyond their contract period intended to remain purely for the income.

Reliance on expatriates imposes obvious costs including salaries, recruitment fees, travel costs and local subsidies. Other potential disadvantages reflect varied medical backgrounds, different quality standards and cultural sensitivities, especially where expatriates speak other languages, which also limits their potential input into training. A key reason for the genesis of the project that initiated this study was country concern over the qualifications and effectiveness of expatriates. The Dean of the FScM bluntly observed in 2003 that overseas-recruited doctors 'don't have a qualification that's worth the paper it's printed on', but confirming this proposition is impossible. At least as early as 1996 in Fiji there was some concern that expatriate SHWs were sometimes challenged by local conditions, as in the case of a group of Chinese doctors 'whose training is allegedly doubtful, their oral English skills were very poor' and who were probably not examined for their skills before leaving China. Moreover, 'patients have also complained about difficulty in communicating with some expatriate doctors, especially Filipino, Burmese and Chinese doctors' (Naidu 1997: 72). Like most abstract claims attached to foreign incompetence, these cannot easily be verified, and expatriate doctors and nurses have been part of Pacific health care systems since their origin. Nonetheless, their supposed failures are part of a perception that the health system is not providing an adequate service, and emphasize that health and health care are cultural phenomena.

While expatriates relieve skill shortages, and in some places make up a significant proportion of the workforce, a crucial advantage of replacement SHWs is that most states have been able to direct them, where necessary, to remote areas where local workers are few. In Fiji and Kiribati, however, Nigerian and Filipino doctors simply refused to work in rural areas, but in the Cook Islands migrant doctors (mostly Burmese) are concentrated in the small and remote northern group, where there are no longer Cook Islands doctors and few local nurses. The two doctors on Tanna Island (Vanuatu) are both Canadian volunteers. Ironically it is precisely in such remote regions, where local people are less likely to be able to speak English (the universal language of migrant health workers, however imperfectly they may speak it themselves), that risks of misunderstanding may occur. In the northern Cook Islands old people especially have difficulty speaking English and tend not to visit a non-English-speaking doctor. In the Marshall Islands too people 'don't feel easily able to communicate with people who speak a different language'. Without indigenous SHWs there is little choice.

Overseas SHWs themselves identified problems, mainly attached to management; many who had come from more sophisticated health care systems were scathing about local inefficiencies and attitudes, 'Pacific time' and lack of resources. Filipina nurses in the Marshall Islands were challenged by what they saw as a more chaotic working environment: the next nurses on shifts did not come, or came late and there was 'chronic absenteeism'. The actual practice of health care posed problems too. They perceived inappropriate cases being sent to emergency and the lack of adequate health education. Overseas nurses in Palau similarly experienced problems: 'nurses and doctors chatting and chewing [betel nut] on the job', 'too many non-nursing duties', 'the high cost of living and the lack of social activities' and the perceived 'lack of professionalism of nurses here, in terms of dress codes and language'. Expatriates were most likely to point to the politics of health and their own weak position in decision-making, somewhat analogous to that of return migrants.

Some degree of self-criticism existed. In Palau several of the expatriate nurses referred to a language barrier and two argued that 'English should be spoken in the workplace'. It is impossible to determine whether frequent references to cultural differences were reflected in the actual delivery of health care, but intermittent comments along the lines of 'a lot of demanding and unfriendly patients tying to belittle me' and 'uncooperative patients', suggest that this may sometimes have been the case. Only one SHW, in Kiribati, was concerned at her own abilities, stating that her limited grasp of the Kiribati language meant that she did not always know what was going on. By contrast one migrant doctor in Palau claimed that he had been so successful that 'I have helped improve the health care system to a satisfactory level comparable with Hawaii'. Others were more sanguine about their efforts and several referred to loosely cultural problems: 'don't speak the language', 'sense of entitlement makes me feel unappreciated', 'the problems of being a non-citizen' and 'the many languages spoken. Hard to understand their English'. Not surprisingly most felt they were coping, though few intended to stay for many years.

The overall impact of overseas SHWs is variable, intangible and ultimately uncertain, but unquestionably they fill a vital gap.

> Chinese doctors are playing a significant role in the provision of medical services in Port Vila and Luganville. While some are probably skilled practitioners, MOH cannot obtain any information on their skills, qualifications and experience. Few develop much capacity in Bislama or English, reducing any potential contribution they can make to the provision of health services . . . Unless suitable and reliable evidence can be provided, recruitment under the aid program should be discontinued. (ADB 2002b: 242)

Vanuatu may have been less well served by expatriate doctors than other states where SHWs have a greater ability to speak English and cultural distances are fewer. Language divides have declined, but continue to influence perceptions of failures in practice. I-Kiribati believe that western-trained doctors are too impersonal and too busy, mainly because they were not emotionally involved with their patient.

> The foreign practitioners do not speak Gilbertese and need a translator. The interaction becomes too complicated and too impersonal, the

> patient feels insecure, uneasy and becomes too resentful towards the medical practitioner. This resentfulness is . . . commonly expressed in the attitude of the patient to prescribed drugs, in that patients fail to take the prescribed medication. (Christensen 1995: 103)

Local SHWs were usually ambivalent about their expatriate colleagues: Frustrated over their superior wages, some found expatriates to be aloof, but most recognised that they usually came from different, often more modern, technical backgrounds and had new and appropriate skills that they could learn from. Costs and cultural differences indicate, however, that this is not necessarily the best way of dealing with sometimes subtle health requirements.

Several expatriates in the Pacific came at some expense from several states, such as Burma and the Philippines, where health care may have been inferior to that of their destinations. Within the Pacific too SHWs tended to be moving from places of greater need to places of lesser need, as Fijians moved to Nauru, Palau and the Marshall Islands, and Solomon Islanders went to the Cook Islands. (These intraregional migrants were particularly well trained and experienced; the loss to Fiji was substantial.) Ironically the lone FSM migrant in Palau originated from one of the exceptionally remote Outer Islands, and had become a nurse 'since the profession was badly needed on the island'. These small fragments of the global care chain display a considerable degree of selectivity in taking health workers to places where salaries are greater and where needs are fewer: the inverse care law revisited.

TO THE ISLANDS: RETURN MIGRATION AND CIRCULATION

If significant return migration of SHWs occurred, sending countries would gain returnees with (usually) enhanced skills and experience, and perhaps also capital and enthusiasm, constituting a positive transfer of knowledge and social capital (unless, as in the first phases of the brain drain, returnees came back with aspirations and demands for technology wholly inappropriate to local needs and budgets). Yet this may only rarely be the case as return migration is becoming less frequent than in earlier years. The extent of global return migration of SHWs has been perceived to be so slight that Kingma (2006) has referred to the 'myth of return'. Migrants are unlikely to be tempted back by a system that they left at least in part because of its perceived shortcomings, though they may return for reasons that have nothing to do with health or because of problems in the destination.

The growth of overseas migrant communities, as the demographic balance shifts, significant income differentials between origin and destination, education overseas (for both migrants and their children) and perceptions of limited opportunities back home have slowed return migration. Superior salaries, facilities and working conditions contribute to new and more congenial workplaces. Children of migrants have been educated in the destination and may have lost some degree of contact with 'home' societies and even linguistic skills, and thus both parents and children would be embarrassed by the prospect, for example, of children returning home unable to speak 'their language'. Intentions to return, most evident before migration, are diluted after departure. While migrants may proclaim anticipated return, that is often the public face of private stability (Macpherson 1994; van Eyck 2004: 27). Indeed, despite often stated intentions, 'it is probably unrealistic to expect more than a tiny fraction of those who have already *escaped* . . . ever to go back. Many will want to go back but only if this want is never put to the test' (Crocombe 1978: 42; my italics). Thus, just one of seven migrant Fijian doctors was open to return, and even then only 'if fired' (Oman 2007). However, intentions are never reality. Duality and ambivalence are as much attached to return as they are to migration.

In the context of migration from Samoa, it has been bluntly stated that 'Polynesian migrants do not return except for visitations, once they are overseas and have attained a degree of security' (Shankman 1976: 96). Few promising economic niches existed, wages were low, children failed to adjust and hierarchical social organization blocked individual aspirations. However, in an era of more skilled migration and greater individualism, overseas education and employment may bring return migrants both status and deference and high relative incomes at home (Marcus 1981: 60). While that might suggest some selectivity towards the return migration of the relatively skilled, in Tonga at least returnees represented a cross-section in terms of age, employment and skill acquisition, and included SHWs (Maron and Connell 2008). Yet in both these two national contexts there were relatively few such skilled return migrants, compared with the number of those who had left.

Although many SHWs had returned, less than 20 percent of them had worked overseas before return and most had never been employed (other than in training contexts) outside the home country. Most returned, often with some degree of reluctance, because they were bonded to do so. Some Pacific island students who take up scholarships overseas do not return, sometimes justified on the grounds that the course was culturally inappropriate to local conditions. Niuean students who had chosen to stay in New Zealand remained because of limited opportunities, low salaries and a generation gap where young graduates perceived themselves as innovative but saw older people as being stuck in their ways and who would give no support to new ideas. Other factors included no job challenges, all the family being resident in New Zealand, the lack of a clear future—including the ability to use acquired skills, lack of mentoring and support, no obvious career path and a feeling that Niue was not going forward (Brunt and Morris-Tafatu 2002: 54). These perspectives, shared by many who have returned, echo the perspectives of those employed in the health sector. Returnees knew only too well what they would be letting themselves in for.

Beyond bonding, social reasons influenced return for both doctors and nurses, including the rather nebulous but constant 'it's my home country', or being with friends and relatives and accompanying a spouse home. For a significant proportion return was a duty as much as an act of free will. Migrants tended to return at key moments in the life cycle—after training or before marriage, for example, or when children had graduated—but often when their parents experienced particular needs. Return is invariably little to do with economics or employment, but is for family reasons, often of households or individuals who had returned to care for aging parents. In other words, many returned not necessarily at times of their own choosing or of their own volition. One nurse returned to Tonga because she had close relatives and friends there and was pleased to be 'able to be with my parents. I was so happy that I was able to look after them until they passed away', while simultaneously she was able 'to raise my daughter in Tonga: looking back I think I made a good decision'. Some parents thus reaped the benefits of their encouragement of employment in the health arena often decades earlier (Chapter 4). Little of this necessarily makes such returnees ideal employees.

Other than those bonded to return (and certainly not all of those), migrants rarely returned out of a desire to work in the health sector. Not all returnees, even those who were previously SHWs, work in the health sector (but because the survey data came from within the sector this proportion cannot be identified). Returning SHWs were particularly likely to establish a business on their return, having accumulated enough savings overseas. Some who had returned to the health sector sought to get into private business or simply 'be a part-time shopkeeper in addition to nursing to earn some extra dollars', or 'set up my own used-clothing business'. Some had achieved that sort of complementarity: 'the main benefit from returning is that I can also work in agriculture and now export beans, capsicum, zucchini and pawpaw' (sixty-one-year-old pharmacist). Business, often by or with their spouse, compensated for salary reductions. The economic rationale for return migration was outside the health sector, giving returnees greater income and a degree of individualism, independence and autonomy, so that many return migrants to the health sector were part of multi-income households. After return to the Cook Islands, for example, as many as half of all men and three-quarters of women moved out of the public sector into the private sector, setting up small businesses. The health sector became mere supplementary employment (Hooker and Varcoe 1999; Rallu 1997; see also Marcus 1981: 60). Incomes in the health sector alone were perceived as inadequate. Returnees returned to the health sector because they could, or should, rather than because they wanted to.

Many of the pleasures of return were detached from any workplace. Lifestyle—which usually meant family and friends, alongside having one's own house and often land, made return tolerable and enjoyable. Land offered security and stability: 'I love the lifestyle here—the freedom and safety, and quietness. It's not safe in New Zealand. I own my own house and land. It's a slower pace of life but I did have some culture shock when I got back [after three years in Auckland] and had to teach myself to speak Cook Islands Maori again'. Overall there was a 'more comfortable pace of life' where it was 'more relaxed—you can do your own thing'. Peace, tranquility and safety were also valued: 'it's more free and there's less stress for bringing up children', whereas 'I was scared of going out in New Zealand'.

Returning was often socially successful, being with family and friends. Many returnees emphasized the climate, safety or more relaxed pace of life, or simply the familiarity of the home country, indicating how crucial social, political and economic stability is to return migration. But that was not for everyone. It could be stultifying. A smaller world may make what was once a home seem more like a prison, bereft of opportunities and excitement and hemmed in by petty restrictions and social controls. Returning to the health sector was similarly unsatisfying.

> If I had not been married I would not have come back but now I am here I want to serve my country. The Ministry of Health has invested a lot in me and so I should work for them. Besides, both me and my husband have good jobs and this is where our relatives and friends are.

One said that returning was good 'for her people and country' but not for her and her family, believing that she could have done better for her extended family had she remained overseas. Duty had overcome desire. Some experienced resentment, where they were paid more than those who had remained, in the tension between new skills, loyalty and local experience (Chapter 5). In Tonga, nurses who had trained overseas had less clinical 'on-the-job' training than locally trained nurses but returned to a higher level than local nurses causing considerable resentment (Cama and Smith 2004). Others who had returned, even out of a sense of duty ('to contribute') found some difficulty in getting work when they returned ('promises' were lost after staff changes, or there were no obvious vacancies) and a lack of welcome (ridicule when overseas graduates made mistakes and old rituals of practice where change was not wanted) and lack of obvious professional development or promotion (Stewart 2004). Such situations encouraged attrition and discouraged potential returnees.

For doctors, with superior pay and status, returning could be easier. A small number of Palauan doctors had returned, but all were over fifty by then. Somewhat ironically they couched this in altruistic terms: 'to do good', 'to help my country people' or 'to participate in nation-building' (as one stated after being away for twenty-eight years). Only one Samoan doctor regretted the decision to return, finding the working conditions in Samoa difficult: 'first, the pay is lousy (overworked and underpaid). Secondly this is my first year as junior registrar and I have been appointed to a post with a lot of responsibilities and been deprived of a lot of sleep'. By contrast, a dentist returning to Tonga observed: 'the knowledge that I gained overseas is invaluable. I have been able to return to work here and start establishing new changes in dental surgery on Tonga. The experience that I gained overseas is good for Tonga's development'. More generally 'my time overseas has made me more open-minded to new ideas and exchanges . . . and just about life in general' (quoted in Maron and Connell 2008). Return migration is not, therefore, without problems; returnees inevitably compare more lavish facilities and wages overseas with those in their homelands and, despite recognising the problems of providing similar salaries and conditions in the Pacific, are nonetheless frustrated by this. Frustrations exist beyond wage levels and facilities.

> I never wanted to come back from Australia because it was not challenging enough but my husband wanted to return. It's not challenging. The case mixes are too few and it is not specialized here. I have to be a generalist and I don't like it. I'd like to go back there again.

Other returnees stressed nepotism and favouritism in island health care systems, alongside the frustrations of being unable to implement changes that worked elsewhere. Indeed, there was not always enthusiasm for the efforts of returnees. As one local Cook Islands doctor stated: 'returning migrant nurses are too old and out of touch, but we will take anything: we have no choice'.

While public health strategy may favour the employment of those with new skills, not everyone wants to see nationals returning and filling scarce and coveted posts (just as expatriates may also be resented). Public statements express the need for stability and return while private practice discourages and mitigates against it—different versions of the duality and ambivalence that are present overseas. In some contexts countries lack adequate absorptive capacity to receive return migrants, and especially to benefit from the new skills and ability to work with new technology that their return might entail.

Those who wanted to leave again, as many did, invariably sought higher wages or superior access to technology and training; the reasons for repeated migration were much like those that first initiated migration (Chapter 5) or were embedded in family needs. Even some of those who were aware they were doing a valuable job, and enjoyed it, found it difficult to balance this with their knowledge of 'higher wages and a better quality of life overseas' that represented a constant lure: 'I want more experience with serious cases and surgical patients', 'Doctors are treated better overseas; here there is corruption and politics, and I'm losing contact with developments in medicine'. This group was usually relatively young. What may bring sometimes repeated migration to an end is that eventually it becomes 'too hard to start again at the bottom' or 'it's too much to change again at my age', alongside a concentration of friends and relatives in one place or the other. Frustrations related to work conditions and lack of recognition of skills and knowledge, which sometimes amounted to at least perceptions of blocked promotion. Those who had been forced to start again at the bottom of the employment hierarchy were particularly annoyed, as others were frustrated by the lack of adequate technology, or resented having had to give up specialized work (Connell 2008a). The 'lack of equipment' and 'stress, pressure, too much work' all affected morale.

Once again, however, many returnees expressed satisfaction at working for the government, because of the prestige, reliability and stability that it provided; they enjoyed their work, had few grievances with the system and found a considerable degree of fulfillment. 'I wanted to pay back the Niuean people and reduce the language barrier that is associated with expatriates, since we understand local values and conditions' and 'I like being able to work with and help my own people'. The health service lends itself to certain forms of satisfaction: 'meeting people from different islands' and 'working closely with the community and getting respect from people' or 'seeing the emergence of new life'. Team-work enthused many. In the upper echelons of the health sector return migrants often valued the particular freedoms and privileges of high-status positions—such as their ability to travel frequently. Working in the public service created a geographical paradox: 'I stay here because there are opportunities for travel overseas'. In six years one health worker had been to conferences or training workshops in nine different countries. Remaining in the Pacific actually enables mobility. Power had its perks and pleasures: 'I was going to return overseas but now I'm in charge'. Others felt they could use their overseas knowledge and much satisfaction was implicit in simply doing a good job and knowing one was contributing. Inevitably frustrations were also attached to 'failures' that were implicit in the very nature of practicing medicine. As many people were concerned about their inability to reduce pain, prevent death or stimulate good practices as had frustrations in the workforce.

In some circumstances qualifications and skills acquired overseas were simply too specialized, most obviously in the smaller states, where a more general multi-skilling characterizes relatively small workforces, and complex procedures are undertaken through overseas referrals. Jane Tupoku exemplified this situation:

> Jane grew up in Niue but completed her final high school year in New Zealand. She then trained there as a nurse since several of her relatives were nurses and she perceived it to be a career that would earn a good living and help her family. After graduation she returned to Niue for two years to fulfill her scholarship bond obligations. She then returned

to New Zealand for a year's midwifery training before again coming back to Niue. At first she enjoyed being back, there were many responsibilities and her New Zealand education meant that she was expected to take on several activities. 'After a bit I no longer had enough patients to retain my interest: there were too many minor mundane things. I used to wonder what they were doing in New Zealand since I was curious about new techniques and ideas. There was not enough interaction here—too few people. You have to get used to sitting. Now I can't work here—my work is much too specialized. In New Zealand I got used to the fast-moving lifestyle—people are over-relaxed and overconfident here. They just take their time and don't seem to care but do it when they feel like it. It's not much of a challenge—I like to be exposed and on my toes, more than just relaxing I want to learn about new technologies. In New Zealand when you need help it's there.' After again fulfilling her bond she went back to New Zealand to work in Wellington, disappointing her parents though she did not intend to go permanently. In New Zealand she enjoyed the lifestyle and people, liked the type and variety of nursing she was doing, interaction with other staff, access to superior resources and the privacy of personal life. Two years later she went to Jeddah in Saudi Arabia, after being contracted by an Auckland agency: 'other nurses had been there and had both positive and negative experiences, the money was great and it was an adventure though we were naïve about it all'. She stayed there seven years, enjoying the work (where she worked in a specialized neonatal unit), the community life and the excellent facilities, despite certain cultural constraints. Briefly she worked alongside another Niuean nurse. Eventually she learned to teach scuba diving all around Egypt, Sinai and elsewhere. After leaving Saudi Arabia she returned to Niue for three months, but then went to Cairns in northern Australia where she could again combine scuba diving with work in a specialized neonatal ICU. There was plenty of work, including work with the Flying Doctor service delivering premature babies, but she eventually found this too quiet and wanted to do a master's degree. Through a magazine advertisement she found that Vancouver was recruiting neonatal nurses and went there since she had heard positive things about the health care system, there was a bigger unit and she could take a further degree. Two years later she returned to Niue in 2004, in the wake of Cyclone Heta that had devastated Niue and destroyed the hospital, and undertook voluntary shifts in the makeshift hospital to relieve the staff. Cyclone Heta made her question why she was in Vancouver, so far from home and family, though she maintained a close connection with family, telephoning a couple of times a week to her parents, e-mailing her brothers and sisters just as frequently and returning from Canada and Saudi Arabia at least once a year. Nonetheless, in 2005 she gained permanent residence in Canada, where she enjoyed the seasons, the 'healthy lifestyle and mentality'. She

> had never married. By 2006, when she had again returned to Niue for her father's funeral, she felt that there would only be one move after Canada and that would be back to Niue. But: 'I can't work here, my nursing is much too specialized, and I'm not inspired here—I would have to get used to sitting around. There is no big picture here, about patients or community, no element of compassion, nursing is just a chore, there is no leadership and inadequate equipment to do a great deal. Eventually the good ones become despondent and leave'. She returned to Canada once more.

Jane exemplified those migrants who have undoubtedly succeeded overseas and, although retaining various close contacts at home, would find it extremely difficult to return, despite family connections and social expectations being orientated towards that. Some careers, and also social lives, are more demanding and fascinating and simply do not exist at home for such 'high-fliers'. Broadly, Jane had become a spiralist, with spiralism 'the progressive ascent of specialists of different skills through a series of higher positions in one or more hierarchical structures, and the concomitant residential mobility through a number of communities during the ascent' (Watson 1964: 147). Return would demand too many social and economic sacrifices and constrained opportunities and, because Jane had siblings who remained at home, there was less pressure on her to return. Even in larger countries some SHWs have simply become too specialized; one neurologist left Fiji knowing there would be insufficient specialized work there after he became a brain surgeon.

Return migration may seem to constitute the worst of both worlds: those who returned to the health sector had been away a short time and gained relatively little in the way of new skills or experience while those who had been away longer and gained valuable skills were unlikely to return to the health sector. Benefits tend to accrue to individuals rather than to the health system. Yet bonding ensures that new skills and young graduates do return, while return is reasonably balanced, and certainly not merely of failures and retirees. The return migration of those with elevated skills, like Jane Tupoku, has been limited, partly because scarce skills cannot necessarily be practiced locally, but more frequently because return migrants are poorly recompensed. Overseas recruitment, whether of ICU nurses (or even footballers), emphasizes this selectivity. Yet even the most established overseas migrants are rarely entirely divorced from home. Return is always possible if unlikely, and remittances flow, unless individuals 'marry out' (to either a member of the host nation or another migrant), a common phenomenon where tertiary education is undertaken overseas.

The principal benefit from return migration should be the transfer of skills and experience acquired overseas, especially into a familiar cultural context. Generally, there is limited evidence that this occurs, as technology often differs and resources are absent, or more simply because return is slight

(Kingma 2006: 201). Equally significant constraints to using new skills, and innovation, rest in rigid hierarchies and uncomprehending and uninterested superiors. Return migrants may be 'agents of change' but conformity is usually more appreciated than change, in workplaces and in local society. It may be that 'it is return migration that slowly changes islands but, wherever and however it occurs, and especially on the smallest islands, migration and change incite resentment, envy, tension and new perceptions of identity' (Connell and King 1999: 18). Many migrants find return difficult, facing lower wages and standards of living, difficulty in establishing businesses and simply culture shock. Optimism can be easily shattered, but while returnees may be few, their impact has led to some gains for health services (through new skills and wider experience) and to the economy through their investment of overseas-generated incomes. Again ambivalence is at the core of Pacific 'cultures of migration', where technical skills must be acquired overseas but dependent families remain at home. Migrants are seemingly forever caught between two worlds, their contributions to national development reduced and their journeys rarely complete (Chapman 1991; Small 1997; Maron and Connell 2008) however much they may sometimes seem to be.

REMITTANCES

While relatively few SHWs may return, they and other skilled migrants make a substantial contribution to the economic well-being of those who remain at home. Creating that income informs many family migration decisions, as households seek to increase incomes by migration and remittance strategies, even by fostering obligations and 'implicit contracts' (Poirine 1997). The use of the money within the home communities means there is always some possibility of return migration. Throughout the Pacific remittances have contributed to national and household development. The gains for both households and countries from remittance flows (especially in Polynesia) indicate that the 'brain drain' of health workers creates some economic gains, especially as over time remittances are more likely to be invested (Connell and Brown 2005). Moreover, remittances have been sustained to a higher level and over longer time periods than has occurred in other parts of the world.

The actual extent of remittances of migrant health workers is largely unknown but, at least in the case of migrant nurses from Samoa and Tonga in Australia, for whom data are available, remittances were sustained at high levels, and thus contributed substantially to the welfare of kin in the home country. Health workers tend to send above-average remittances over longer time periods, perhaps because women were more reliable remitters, or because they were more altruistic. Where households have invested in human capital and the choice of occupation was linked to the possibility of migration, then individuals are more generous and reliable remitters, and there is the greatest propensity to return (Brown and Connell 2004, 2006; Connell and Brown 2005). Though there are no contemporary data, remittances probably remain at similar high levels, and the same conclusion probably applies to other skilled migrants.

Remittances are particularly important in the smaller states of Polynesia, and in the more remote islands of all states, where they play an increasingly important role in household and national economies as a significant part of disposable income. Remittances are primarily used for consumption and welfare objectives, including improved housing and some community goals (such as water tanks and churches), alongside education, and contribute to subsequent human resource development, sustaining social networks and creating social capital (Grieco 2003). Education is highly valued, both generally and for the development of specific skills, to create human capital for potential migration. Even with imperfect knowledge, households consciously make decisions in favour of the quantity and quality of education of children that boost their chances for migration and thus the supply of remittances (Brown and Connell 2004). Remittances are subsequently used for various forms of investment, especially into stores and transport businesses, stimulating entrepreneurial and trading activity, increasing the extent of formal sector employment and creating multiplier effects (Connell and Brown 2005). Successful development of small businesses provides some incentive for those who have sent remittances to return home and manage those businesses. Migration and remittances thus stem from and contribute both directly and indirectly to various forms of capital formation.

The role of SHWs is of some economic significance. Overall remittances are positive and satisfying for households but insufficient to influence national development goals. While the remittances generated by SHWs may have been earned partly because of the training they acquired in local schools and tertiary health institutions they do not return there. Education (including scholarships) is mainly in the public sector, remittances return to households and the private sector (other than churches and some village projects) and only indirectly provide any benefit to the education and health system that produced the migrants. They may lead to greater expenditure on medical services, take some pressure off the public sector and boost household incomes enabling some SHWs to stay, but that cannot easily be demonstrated. Though the remittances from SHWs may be substantial they do not directly compensate for the skill drain. The economic future of several states partly hinges on the continued flow of remittances, and hence on continuity of migration, a situation not necessarily more difficult where migration becomes more selective by skills. The possibility of blocked migration in the future, a situation ever present in public debate (Macpherson 1992; Shankman 1993; World Bank 2006), emphasizes potential problems especially within a 'culture of migration' that is an important element of household and national social and economic systems.

DESKILLING AND BRAIN LOSS?

> Things change. There's no live happily ever after.
>
> (Tongan nurse in Australia, quoted in Fusitu'a 2000: 66)

Social costs are attached to migration as families are fragmented across and between countries, especially when female nurses migrate alone overseas. Separation usually does little for family harmony despite the transnational corporation of kin being an accepted basis for migration. Many households of SHWs have found real difficulties in becoming re-established in overseas destinations in terms of employment, accommodation or simply cultural differences. There may also be benefits, beyond income generation; many Fijian nurses moved to the Marshall Islands to escape disintegrating, unfulfilling relationships and achieved greater happiness (Rokoduru 2008). That may be exceptional; meanwhile other long-distance relationships collapse. Though many of those who have gone to UAE or the regional United Kingdom have flourished, not all migrants have made smooth, satisfying transitions between places and social contexts.

What happens to SHWs in their destinations is of considerable importance. In recent years those who have been actively recruited have undoubtedly used their skills effectively in destinations as diverse as Dubai and Dunedin, have received salaries much greater than available at home and contributed enormously to health systems. Where migrants made individual decisions the outcomes are less positive and the evidence of success more ambivalent. In the United States, many Micronesians, Fijians and probably other islanders, some of whom were SHWs at home, work as poorly paid, unskilled caregivers in nursing homes (Scott 2003; Marshall 2004; Connell and Voigt-Graf 2006). Many Fijians without formal qualifications are working in nursing homes in Australia and New Zealand. Other Pacific islanders have worked temporarily in such contexts. Many nurses have migrated as partners rather than workers, and often took up 'temporary' unskilled work in factories, or were needed to support families, before eventually seeking to get their qualifications recognised and take up nursing positions. Some, in every destination, never succeeded.

> A Senior Staff Nurse at Vaiola Hospital Mele took six months leave in the United States, where she visited friends and relatives and did relief work in housekeeping and palliative care. She was able to earn a little

> extra income to complement the amount she earned from her role as a nurse in Tonga. (Maron 2001: 46)

Niuean nurses in New Zealand were similarly unrecognised and many sought unskilled work in factories or were employed as nurse aides in rest homes. From a large sample of Pacific nurses in New Zealand, most of whom were Samoan or Tongan, those who were not active nurses were working in rest homes and residential care, having failed to have their qualifications recognised or registered, and so earned lower incomes (Koloto 2003: 47, 87–90). Not only were nursing skills—even unrecognised—effectively discarded, but when nurses again took up nursing they tended to be in the least skilled areas. Pacific islander nurses in New Zealand mainly work in continuing care, particularly of the elderly, and very few were in management; compared with nurses as a whole they were disproportionately likely to be employed in public hospitals, rest homes or residential care (Koloto 2003). Whether in Australia, New Zealand or the United States, nurses were working in the least skilled and strategically important areas. Migration has been no great success story in the short term here, other than in its ability to keep the health systems of metropolitan states functioning. However, as the number of Pacific islander nurses in nursing associations in New Zealand alone indicates, let alone doctors and those elsewhere, large numbers of migrants are at the very least productively employed as SHWs overseas.

Not all migrants continue as SHWs after migration for various reasons. A substantial number of Tongan nurses in Australia gave up nursing partly because their qualifications were not recognised (and they needed jobs immediately to pay off debts and rent etc.), thus 'finding work was often a matter of subsistence and the fact that many "fell into" nursing again, a function of familiarity rather than vocational passion' (Fusitu'a 2000: 60). Work was sometimes distant from homes, new family structures posed different demands and jobs such as taxi-driving offered a flexibility absent from health. Despite their considerable diversity few had achieved substantial upward mobility within the health system; some were disappointed that they had not achieved greater success but none sought to return to Tonga. Several had children who did not speak Tongan and would have been unfamiliar and acutely disadvantaged there. Several stated that the jobs they had now had no equivalent in Tonga, which might have been 'a guiltless way of saying no' to return (Fusitu'a 2000: 72). For many the simple fact that the majority of their own families now lived in Sydney largely negated that option.

Few SHWs overseas, however successful they had or had not been, therefore sought to return, with many Tongans in New Zealand staying because of their own, their partner's or their children's access to higher wages, superior education and professional support. Several doctors professed a wish to return to 'give something back to my home country' or to 'help the local situation' but return had been indefinitely postponed, as 'the time was not right'. Only two of twenty-three Tongan nurses in New Zealand intended to return during their working lifetime, perhaps not an indictment of the poor working environment, low pay and limited educational opportunities for themselves and their children that had caused them to migrate, but an indication of how permanent migration had become.

Where migration was the primary goal, skilled work was sometimes abandoned. One Fijian doctor had become a shopkeeper in New Zealand; he used his status as a doctor 'to acquire a New Zealand medical licence but chose to become a shopkeeper instead. He said that his career mattered less to him than the fact that a variety of tertiary educational opportunities were now accessible to his children' (Naidu 1997: 69). The survey methodology excluded other possible examples. Nonetheless, this may have been a rare example, as Indo-Fijian doctors have characteristically remained doctors overseas and been particularly successful. However, even for some of the most skilled, migration may have little directly to do with health issues.

While migration is a loss to Pacific sending countries the gains in destinations were often muted. Though there is minimal information on those SHWs who simply failed to practice at all in their destinations, for many who were practicing, their positions were often below those at home. Not only were SHWs, especially nurses, migrating internationally within the context of the 'inverse care law', but they were often being at least partially deskilled as the outcome of that process. The result was brain waste. Islanders themselves are conscious that their knowledge, experience and skills constitute a loss to their home countries, which most seek to remedy on a temporary or permanent basis by return or on a continuing basis through remittances.

CONCLUSION: FROM THE ISLANDS? THE WIDER BRAIN DRAIN

> Our skilled health practitioners are return aid to New Zealand.
>
> (Bob Talagi, Niue, June 2003)

Retaining SHWs in small island states is particularly difficult, since some skills are of limited local utility, salary differentials with overseas are greatest for skilled workers, who may be bored and dissatisfied with local employment, and working conditions are challenging. At least as importantly, however, their extended families are interested in migration. The consequence is a brain or skill drain, even a brain waste, that emphasizes how education represents a critical investment in human capital. The outcome is less well-satisfied health needs, and reduced morale amongst those who have remained, as working conditions deteriorate. Wards are closed, waiting lists and times lengthen, examinations are more cursory or complicated by new cultural differences. Large proportions of budgets, already thinly spread, are directed to referrals and replacements. Because of the necessity for appropriate training, it is more difficult to substitute for (or transfer from elsewhere in the public service) absent skills in the health workforce.

Yet even in such a critical area it remains difficult to go much beyond anecdote in analysis of the consequences of migration. There is simply inadequate data for a cost-benefit analysis that elegantly balances education costs, remittances, social costs and so on. The number of strikes or threatened strikes in the health sector have increased in recent years, but that can have many causes, while perhaps selective fragments of data, as in Samoa, point to situations where 40 percent of all doctors are beyond retirement age and 'personnel shortages make it difficult for staff to take leave and go overseas for training' (World Bank 1998: 19). There, and more generally, health resources seem stretched alarmingly, in downward spirals and vicious circles.

Pacific island countries have been unable to restructure and modernise health care systems, or provide incomes and broader working conditions, comparable with those in developed countries. The intensifying global structure of demand and recruitment ensures that relatively poor island states continue to experience a steady migration of SHWs. That skill drain only belatedly provides some gains through human capital transfers (with return migration), remittances and the investments of returnees. Individuals and households have gained from migration, rather more than wider society and economy, except in the destinations. Remote areas particularly have lost, perhaps ultimately worsening the welfare and bargaining position of those places. Migrants remain intricately enmeshed in social networks that place them within a complex transnational corporation of kin and ensure that however long they have been away they have essentially 'gone away without leaving' (Nietschmann 1979: 22). Their skills may be largely lost to the islands but their economic contribution, scarcely muted over time, is a substantial one. Yet the evidence that exists, fragmented and superficial though it often is, indicates that Pacific island states, like other source areas of migrant health workers, on balance are towards the losing end of a global care chain that benefits metropolitan recipient countries at the expense of the sources. There is a consensus that migration is not overspill but a definite loss, with clear negative outcomes that are both economic and health related, limiting progress towards healthy islands and possibly even resulting in a regression from that status. Policies and practices to remedy such issues have been widely sought.

7 A Policy Perspective?

A well-established structure and a dual culture of migration have become established in the Pacific. Skilled health workers have moved to take advantage of superior wages and salaries, training and research opportunities and working conditions for themselves, and to better the lifestyles of their children and extended families, through education, social change and remittances. Migration is likely to continue, especially where there have been structural reforms that reduce public sector employment, wages and salaries remain unequal, working conditions are difficult and kin are increasingly overseas where demand is increasing. Policies that redress such diverse circumstances have proved difficult for small island states, while governments have rarely sought to intervene in the process of international migration. Indeed, once concerned over the diverse costs of migration, islanders, from individuals and households to extended families and national governments, are increasingly likely to seek out new migration opportunities.

A perceived shortage of SHWs is common to all island states, though this has been partially remedied by various strategies (including retaining staff after retirement age and recruiting from overseas). Yet even defining shortage is challenging: vacancy rates are of value, but defining the staffing establishment is difficult, where nurses may undertake the more 'invasive therapy' of drips and drains, and bed-making and store maintenance are devolved to others. Politicians, bureaucrats, SHWs and patients differ in their assessments of needs and unions invariably claim that their members are overworked (and underpaid). In an ideal world national and regional training facilities would develop appropriate numbers of skilled people who would deliver effective services. But in many island states failures of governance, broadly the inadequate delivery of services (whether health, education, transport etc.), have been key constraints to development, and particularly to long-term human resources development.

Within countries there is some ambivalence towards migration. In Melanesia there are perceptions of excess migration to urban centres and often draconian policies directed to reversing this, notably in PNG but also in

Fiji and Vanuatu (Connell and Lea 2002; Connell 2003c). Policies that focus on decentralization and regional development are largely things of the past (Connell 1987a) as states exercise a more limited role in policy formation. That limited role is even more evident for international migration. Few countries have actually sought to address migration directly, largely because it is seen as impossible to prevent (or even discourage). Freedom of movement is perceived as a human right, previously taken advantage of by other workers and kin, while policymakers themselves are prone to migration.

Not all countries have sought to prevent migration; elsewhere, some, like the Philippines and Cuba, purposefully export workers, including health workers, either to earn valuable foreign exchange (mainly through remittances) or fulfill avowedly humanitarian goals. Pacific states have been increasingly drawn to similar policies (see the following), and several have trained workers for overseas employment, notably in the Marine Training Schools of Tuvalu and Kiribati. On several occasions Tuvalu has drawn attention to the need for new migration outlets because of the difficulties of sustaining populations in a small, densely populated island state, with few resources, alongside the problems of absorbing return migrants (Connell 2003b: 94–95). Many states are currently interested in increased volumes of migration, at least for unskilled workers, so that discouraging the movement of skilled workers—and only one particular group of them—is both difficult and even inequitable. Several states have expressed particular concerns, such as the loss of skilled labour (including nurses and army personnel), the breaching of bonds by scholarship holders or, in the case of Niue, particularly extensive migration. For the past quarter of a century governments have not sought to curb the emigration of skilled and unskilled workers. They are unlikely to do so in the future.

POLICY OPTIONS

Mobility is often enshrined in national constitutions, and it is sometimes argued that this should not be constrained, particularly for skilled professionals with valuable skills. An open international market is said to offer efficiency and economic gains. However, while there are gains in economic efficiency at an aggregate level those gains are localized in receiving countries, and in sending countries the benefits are much less evident (Chapter 6). As the evidence of costs to national health (and economic and social) systems has mounted there has been a greater interest in developing policies and mechanisms to diminish and mitigate the impacts of migration. All Pacific island states have some options for increasing the numbers of SHWs, reducing attrition, improving retention and reducing the overseas flow. Yet in a context of weak public policy formation, stemming the flow of SHWs, or even increasing the benefits from that flow, is hard to achieve.

Recruitment

Fewer people are now being attracted to health careers. Despite the possibility of migration, wages and conditions in the public health sector are increasingly seen as deterrents to entry and other sectors are perceived as more attractive. In the Cook Islands, for instance, in the 1950s and 1960s the health sector was extremely attractive, but by the 1980s the national economic focus had shifted from agriculture towards tourism and business and even health scholarships were perceived as less prestigious (Connell 2005). Potential employees now witness the frustrations of health workers, there are other job options and a career in health has less prestige and income benefits than it once had. In some places nursing is seen as a dirty, dangerous and difficult, perhaps even degrading, job, though medicine retains its lure, and some Pacific islanders are now disdainful of a career in health.

Nonetheless, a basic solution involves creating more places for those who wish to become SHWs, even though attrition rates are high and the cost of training is considerable. In several states a familiar bureaucratic response has been 'train more people' and 'train them here'. The recruitment of adequate numbers of trainees, and creating more places is not straightforward. Several countries lack the capacity to train substantially larger numbers. Failures of recruitment reflect education in high schools, which may be inadequate for high school graduates to be confident of a career in the health system (or for the health system to take them on). In Palau, where that was common, the MOH launched a 'Bridging Program' where high school graduates were hired as nursing assistants for four hours a day and given extra classes to enable them to qualify (Miho 2007). Effective recruitment or 'outreach' programmes in schools may, however, only be successful after the restructuring of the wage structures and working practices of SHWs, particularly nurses.

Some countries have thus thrown the net wider. Many states have, at least in part, a 'pseudoshortage', where former nurses and other SHWs are there but are unwilling to work at the prevailing conditions. In the Cook Islands former workers have been encouraged to return from retirement, but not entirely successfully. A number of nurses came back but 'several of these nurses are set in their ways and have difficulty being good team members or carrying out a full day's work' (SAGRIC International 2000: 27). A contributory factor to the loss of SHWs in the region (through attrition) has been the enforcement of a mandatory retirement age. In both Fiji and Samoa there has been a policy of employing retired local medical officers on a yearly contract basis to fill vacancies. In Samoa, nurses and doctors are the only public servants who can go beyond the retirement age as long as they are functioning effectively. Kiribati has kept many doctors in service past retirement age.

Conventionally the health workforce has been recruited from immediate school and tertiary education leavers. Tonga has both sought to recruit previously 'trained staff that have had families and are ready to return to the workforce' (Tonga 2000), while also accepting mature students up to the age of forty-five. Similarly the Fiji School of Nursing has abandoned its established policy of only recruiting up to an age limit of twenty-five. Such 'established' residents, with families, are less likely to be interested in migration.

Throughout the Pacific most, often almost all, nurses are women. Many countries have not begun to go beyond these gender stereotypes to consider the more active recruitment of men, as there has been considerable cultural opposition. One survey of Fijian nurses, 97 percent of whom were female, found that 46 percent opposed increasing the intake of males, despite there being a shortage of labour, because the few male nurses climbed the career structure particularly quickly (Fong 2003). The low wages paid to nurses are at least partly a result of the gendered division of labour and concentration of women in these professions, within a loosely male sphere of curing and a female sphere of caring (Leckie 2000), hence a shift towards the recruitment of male nurses might even enhance, though it should not, the possibility of better earnings, and higher retention rates.

Some states have sought preferential recruitment of nurses especially from rural areas and outlying islands, since they are more likely to stay and work there, but this has proved difficult since such potential recruits are often locationally disadvantaged by poorer education levels. Some countries, such as Samoa, have found all too often that 'it just doesn't keep people there—it's a passport out; they don't want to go back'.

Training Locally

Throughout the region locally trained SHWs are more likely to stay (and may have also acquired more appropriate skills) than those trained overseas, hence training programmes have increasingly been located within countries, and upgrading of skills been done by migrant educators rather than learned by migrant SHWs. Since the early 1990s in Samoa there was some slowing of the migration of doctors partly as a result of a decision to have all training of medical officers at the FScM, because of the perception that training there was more appropriate and cheaper than in New Zealand, and 'there was a lower propensity for graduates to emigrate to rim countries relative to graduates of rim country institutions' (World Bank 1994: 322). In-country training is invaluable for the retention of SHWs, but is not always possible and is inadequate without other changes in health systems.

Countries have adapted medical curricula to local needs, because of the obvious relevance and because it potentially reduces the employability of local graduates elsewhere. In the 1990s the FScM developed a Primary Practitioner course, whose graduates were not intended to be internationally marketable, and later developed a master's programme. Increasingly however, as global health trends have tended to converge, for example with the rise of NCDs in developing countries, the need for a distinct curriculum has declined. Moreover, both in the Caribbean and within the Association of South-East Asian Nations (ASEAN), there has been a move to ensure a similar curriculum across the region, to enable the regional accreditation and mobility of health workers. As public policy has moved away from nationalist positions, constraining mobility through a place-specific curriculum is unlikely to be acceptable.

Bonding

The single most important policy to have slowed migration, and a rare direct approach, has been bonding, which has had considerable success in many states in bringing people back to their home countries after education and training overseas (Chapter 6). Bonding also occurs at a significant time in the life cycle, coinciding for some with the start of family life and the possibility of establishing local family roots. Everywhere bonding implies a sense of duty, and emphasizes costs, even though skilled workers have tended to leave at the end of the bond period (usually equivalent to the two or three years that have been spent overseas). While it has been detested and resisted, when few other skilled workers are similarly directed, and the regulations often broken, it has been invaluable, as much for the practice of return as in the inculcation of notions of duty and loyalty.

Wages, Salaries and Employment

Wages and salaries have almost universally been seen as inadequate. Frequent strikes indicate that raising salaries is particularly difficult where budgets are small and relativities within (and beyond) the public sector constrain increases. In Samoa, in response to a strike threat, the Minister of Health commented that nurses had more claim to a pay increase than others in the public service: 'The duties and hardships of nursing are unique to the nursing profession. If the nurses successfully negotiate a T$9,045 (US$3,800) per annum starting salary for those with a Diploma in Nursing, all other Diploma holders think they are entitled to the same salary' (quoted in *Samoa Observer*, 7 May 2000). Although the World Bank has recommended that 'Doctors should be paid at least as well as members of other professions (e.g. lawyers) and may need to be given additional allowances and bonuses, depending on labor market conditions and options for emigration' (World Bank 1994: 30, 324), implementing such a strategy would precipitate wage inflation and broad perceptions of inequity.

Marginally improving wages could never be enough to significantly reduce the demand for migration, given the substantial wage and salary differences between sending and receiving countries. Where two-thirds of health budgets are already absorbed by labour costs, it is impossible to pay international 'market' salaries comparable with those in metropolitan states.

Movements towards superior salary scales might threaten the achievement of decentralization and PHC.

The ability to work in the usually better resourced and remunerated private sector is a disincentive to migration, though enabling such opportunities has been resisted in several states where it is seen to divert doctors away from public responsibilities and areas of particular need. At least in Fiji, 'it seems that once a doctor resigns from the government he [sic] becomes an outcast' in that the public sector no longer sought to take any advantage of their skills (Naidu 1997: 77). More recently there has been a more pragmatic approach enabling some fluidity (see the following), but getting the right balance between being able to work in both sectors without disadvantaging either is difficult.

A Workplace Package?

Most SHWs cite wages, multiple workplace problems, often centred on uncertain career progression, inadequate support (in a personal and technical sense) and a simple lack of appreciation as sources of dissatisfaction. Policies aimed at retention therefore require a package of working conditions, rather than ad hoc piecemeal measures. Such policy combinations have been elaborated many times, developing themes first raised by Gish (1971) and Mejia, Pizurki and Royston (1979) in the 1970s, by organizations such as the Commonwealth Secretariat (2001) and WHO (2006b). Improved working conditions (better wages and access to technology, cleaner hospitals, adequate supplies, more amenable shift systems, support and guidance etc.) improve morale and slow migration. Such changes can be costly and require subtle and responsive management. Various attempts to develop some forms of package have occurred in the Pacific.

In Fiji a series of attempts have been made to discourage resignation and improve the health system, including, over a ten-year period in the 1990s, implementation of an improved salary structure, sponsored postgraduate training opportunities at the FScM, continuing education programmes, attachments and twinning opportunities with overseas hospitals and locum practice for government doctors when they are on leave (to earn some extra money). Such attempts at change also included private practice for specialists and consultants using government facilities after hours (so that they too could earn extra money), upgrading of subdivisional hospitals and health facilities (with more doctor positions being made available), improvement in the supply of drugs, stores and biomedical equipment to facilitate service delivery (and enable doctors to concentrate more on their key functions), decentralization of health management (giving peripheral staff more decision-making responsibility and accountability for their actions) and more transparency in staff promotions and transfers. No review was undertaken of the specific success of implementing these policies, either collectively or individually, or even to see if they were implemented, but one conclusion was drawn that 'the above incentives, though comprehensive, seem to be largely ineffective as doctors continue to resign at the same rate through these years' (Tuqa 1999: 9). Tuqa therefore concluded that doctors should be seen as a special case within the public service, because of the long sustained nature of the shortage problem, its complexity and the socioeconomic costs of the shortage, and should receive substantially better remuneration within a new administrative structure that gave greater attention to promotion structures and training opportunities. The 2000 coup, however, intervened and renewed migration occurred.

Flexibility has not always been present for work practices. Offering part-time work to presently unemployed workers could be invaluable but some Public Service Commissions, such as that of Fiji, prevent any part-time work. Samoa has introduced a 'flexi-roster' that enables nurses to work at times appropriate to them as long as they work for eight hours. Promotion opportunities are few in small island state bureaucracies, currently often doubly so where younger workers rose very quickly in the post-independence years, blocking opportunities for those who sought to follow, especially where few workers are required. Island states, such as Solomon Islands, clearly 'cannot afford to keep expanding the bureaucracy to create posts at will for the sake of promotions' (Ramo 1991: 270), though a transparent promotion structure is invaluable, to ensure that health workers are not doubly disadvantaged. Even objectivity and impartiality are hard to achieve where interpersonal relations are particularly close as they are in the smaller states like Kiribati, and where individuals are able to manipulate systems (Bakeea 1991: 261–262). Annual review of salaries, a clear career structure with opportunities for ongoing training and delegation of responsibilities at least boost the morale of those for whom opportunities of promotion are poor (Bakeea 1991: 256).

External agencies have recommended similar packages. To slow migration of doctors from Samoa the World Bank recommended that the Samoan government should raise their pay and benefits through the 'judicious granting of allowances over and above base salaries which link the rewards of doctors to work loads and health system needs' and argued that the exact nature of such a system would have to be determined empirically and 'be related to future options for migration' so that the actual remuneration of professionals (including doctors) working long hours and on night shifts would not be limited by reference to salary points in the public service but be related to actual scarcities and needs (World Bank 1994: 336). That complex and detailed formulation is indicative both of the concern attached to migration and of the complexities of actually resolving the situation. Samoa never sought to put such complexity into practice. Nonetheless, perhaps unsurprisingly, the World Bank later again concluded that Samoa needed a human resource plan that would:

> provide incentives that will improve staff performance, including attractive salaries, benefits such as in-service training programs linked to salary increments, well-structured career development paths and performance based rewards and sanctions for improper referral. Health professionals must be given remuneration packages including a benefit package and bonuses should be based on labor market conditions. (World Bank 1998: 19)

Once again, what was being recommended was logical but complex, and almost certainly incapable of being monitored even if acted upon within a weak bureaucracy.

Ironically one of the features of small island state bureaucracies most attractive to government workers are certain perks, such as the possibility of going to overseas (or local) courses and conferences that provide an enjoyable break and experience, a means of acquiring sometimes substantial per diem payments, access to 'the latest fashions and electronic goods' and considerable prestige by being selected to go and being treated with respect in the destination. The flexibility that enables more senior bureaucrats to go on such courses makes management less effective as 'things come to a standstill while they are away' (Ramo 1991: 281), further affecting the morale of those who remain in place. Perks come at a cost, but they can be invaluable.

'CHANGING THE RULES': NURSE PRACTITIONERS AND MEDICAL ASSISTANTS

It is no accident that poorly paid, low status nurses are more likely to wish to migrate than doctors, and much more likely to resign. At the same time, as in Samoa, the lack, and loss, of doctors has been more pronounced than that of nurses. This loss has inhibited the performance of the health care system (especially in more remote areas), and the loss of doctors has placed greater pressure on nurses and increased the demand for, and role of, nurses. In several states the response has been to develop a system of nurse practitioners who play an intermediate role between doctors and nurses.

Policies and practices that upgrade nursing skills so that nurses undertake a series of tasks hitherto undertaken by doctors have been successful in various places, with the dual advantage of relieving hard-pressed doctors and giving greater job satisfaction to nurses, especially where they provide some curative services and receive additional status, prestige and salaries. Such a strategy better uses the time and skills of both doctors and nurses. While superior training improves the status of nurses, it also makes their qualifications more transferable.

As in some other countries, the role of nurse practitioner was introduced by the MOH in Fiji to improve access to adequate health care in remote areas, where doctors were few. Nurse practitioners were highly successful in rural service delivery (where they had to be based) and in boosting their status (Usher and Lindsay 2003). By 2007 nurse practitioners had replaced doctors and medical assistants in almost half the nation's seventy-six health centres. In Vanuatu and Kiribati nurse practitioners are established members of health care teams. The growth of Vanuatu's Nurse Practitioner Program, that began in 1983, by bridging the gap between nurses and doctors again enabled more effective delivery of rural services, despite inadequate working facilities (such as lighting and transport), shortage of staff and drugs and limited supervision (Tsiaban 2002). There have been disappointments: in the Solomon Islands many nurse practitioners quickly contracted urban marriages to avoid being posted to remote areas.

The lack of SHWs in most rural areas has also meant instituting community health workers (health assistants or nurse aides), with a limited training for work at the local level. This confers prestige on participants, contributes to bridging the gap between the hospitals and the villages and enables some focus on preventative health care. However, inadequate management and mentoring, poor education standards, inadequate supplies, misdiagnosis and patient preferences for 'superior' skills have blunted their effectiveness and seen them bypassed.

The rise of nurse practitioners, and of community health workers, has also been resented by some, notably doctors, who see this as an erosion of their privileges and authority. Demarcation disputes, prestige and privilege hamper innovation. In the Cook Islands, from the 1990s, nurse practitioners were trained for work in the remote northern islands, a system that worked well (assisted by salary bonuses), until for political reasons doctors were sent there. There was subsequent feeling that the overseas doctors who went there (from India and later Burma) were less effective than the nurse practitioners, who had then been redeployed and were unable to use their superior skills. When Tonga developed a new category of Health Officer, trained in a limited two-year course within Tonga, and who largely ran rural health centres or worked in hospital outpatient wards, their replacement of doctors produced controversy: 'public perceptions of their competence have been less than fully favorable' (World Bank 1994: 322). Typically 'the mirage of "quality medicine" tends to displace legitimate demands for simple but competent and readily available service delivery in the rural areas', hence, when the Samoan MOH similarly sought to create a new 'medical assistant', intermediate between a doctor and nurse, members of parliament who had hospitals in their districts resisted this in their demand for fully certified doctors, so contributing to 'credential inflation', public dissatisfaction and urban migration (Hoadley 1980: 452). Overcoming such perceptions and responses is as difficult as the provision of comparable services and staff in the regions.

STIMULATING RETURN MIGRATION

The growing extent of international migration in recent years, and especially the loss of skilled workers, has resulted in global attention being given to the potential for utilizing the skills of overseas migrants, even on a temporary basis, and to encouraging return migration. Diasporas and remittances have assumed new importance (Faist 2008) in a context of aid fatigue. Given limited permanent return migration, temporary return is increasingly held out as offering more development potential. Pacific countries, even where the migration of skilled workers has been significant, have no strategies or policies for benefiting from such migrants, though many of them are at least rhetorically anxious to support their home countries, send remittances and occasionally contribute directly to health practice (Chapter 2). Where SHWs have returned it has rarely been easy for them to become effectively reintegrated without some local resentment and their own dissatisfaction (Chapter 6), so that even developing policies that encourage return may receive limited local sympathy.

A number of countries have partly dissociated themselves from overseas migrants, on the grounds that they have abandoned their home countries (even if they send remittances), and national policies should be directed towards benefiting those who remain. The Fiji government once tended to regard emigrants as 'traitors' and some policies effectively punish return migrants, for example, where returning nurses had to start at the bottom of the salary scale. While this might have discouraged the temporary migration of nurses in the first place, it certainly discouraged return migration. In 2006 the policy was replaced but returnees still started on a salary one step below when they left. Most island states are unlikely to be able to provide adequate opportunities in the health sector alone to attract back skilled migrants, and it may be necessary to encourage investment opportunities, or provide housing loans, to encourage return migration (Connell and Brown 2005). Addressing the interests of migrants, returnees and residents is not necessarily incompatible but appropriate policies are yet to be developed.

MANAGED MIGRATION: MEETING THE MARKET?

In this century a more controversial and seemingly contradictory response to health worker shortages has emerged. Island states have recognised that it is essential to produce more SHWs than predicted local needs since at least some will migrate. Following 'the Philippines model'—a deliberate strategy of producing significantly more health workers on the basis that many will migrate, and others resign, and migration can be state-regulated enabling economic benefits through remittance flows—such 'overproduction' may be potentially valuable since there are economic advantages from overseas recruitment.

The 'Philippines model' has centred on the assumptions that many SHWs will migrate anyway, most training is in the private sector, there are enough SHWs in the Philippines and remittances are greater than the cost of the training, so there is a net national benefit. Small Caribbean states have more recently sought a context for 'managed migration' that would take the region closer to the regulated Philippines system, and so counter the skill drain: 'a long-term and more sustainable solution would be to enlarge training facilities to meet the expanding demand in labour importing countries' (Nurse 2004: 4). In 2002 a regional health strategy was endorsed that planned for the emigration of a certain proportion of the region's health professionals, and would enable the rotating and short-term migration of others. New nursing schools have been established, primarily to produce nurses for export, as in St. Vincent, with the majority going to work for hospital partners in the United States, who would pay for the entire training cost (Connell 2007e), but with constraints on how long nurses might stay overseas before returning, a situation that amounted to contract labour migration. However, there are doubts over the general willingness of recruiting countries to enter into long-term and expensive contracts, hence the outcomes of the Caribbean experiment are yet to be examined. In the past, efforts to secure compensation for losses have foundered for many reasons, including rejection of the specificity of health worker migration, the impossibility of estimating costs and shifts of workers between the public and private sectors. Previous consideration of this, more than a quarter of a century ago (Gish and Godfrey 1979), was rejected as too idealistic. It probably remains so.

In 2005 the ADB and Commonwealth Secretariat commissioned a study of the potential for a regional training institution for nurses. The study suggested that Pacific states might collectively support a training programme for about 150–200 nurses, that might be established in conjunction with a similar facility in one of the major destinations, and negotiate with one or more destination governments over accreditation and regulations for hiring. The economic assumption was that 'the private benefits and costs [would] be split between the nurses and their families and the government, with the government receiving taxes and perhaps training fees paid by the nurses', with remittances significantly outweighing establishment and training costs (Duncan 2005: 3; ADB 2005). It was assumed both that current Pacific nurses found it difficult to get overseas employment and that there was 'considerable potential for increases in the number of people [to be] trained as nurses and willing to work overseas' (Duncan 2005: 4). However, for nurses from most states overseas accreditation is not now particularly difficult, and the supply of adequately educated high school leavers is limited.

For unskilled workers the outwards orientation is particularly evident. In 2007 five Pacific island states (Kiribati, Tuvalu, Samoa, Tonga and Vanuatu) established guest worker schemes for agricultural workers to spend a period of up to seven months in a year working in New Zealand, and most states have requested Australia to provide similar opportunities (Hammond and Connell 2009; World Bank 2006). The 'export' of semi-skilled workers is yet to be organized. However, Hans Keil, the associate Trade Minister for Samoa and the principal Pacific Islands Forum Secretariat negotiator with the EU, has discussed the possibility of new employment opportunities in Europe:

> We want to open up job opportunities for our people. We are asking for three years and these are not unskilled workers, we want semi-skilled at the moment. That includes care givers, hospital workers, construction workers, rugby players, security officers, hospitality workers. These are people who will go up there to better their skills and then come back to use those skills in developing our countries. Hopefully it will be approved and as the years go by, we will include doctors and other professionals. At the moment we've got seafarers from the Pacific who are employed all over the world. (Quoted in *Islands Business*, June 2007: 23)

Kiribati has sought to extend the seafarer programme to cover nurses, and both Tonga and Samoa would like to train more professionals than can be employed locally (Ware 2005: 445–446). In 2007 the Solomon Islands was considering the possibility of establishing a Caregiver Training Program, with Canadian funding to supply the Canadian market, and a year later the University of the South Pacific, based in Fiji and covering twelve island states, was intending to introduce a caregiver course.

Through its aid programme Australia established a multi-country Australia-Pacific Technical College in 2007 to 'provide internationally recognized Australian-standard vocational training' to increase the pool of skilled workers in targeted industry sectors, where skills were perceived to be lacking in the region. These included tourism/hospitality, automotive, manufacturing, construction and electrical trades and health and community services, initially based in Vanuatu, Fiji, Samoa and PNG, but with the first students also coming from the Solomon Islands, Nauru, Kiribati and Tonga. It aimed to produce three thousand graduates in four years. By 2008 courses had begun in all but health and community services, which were scheduled for 'the near future'. The stated benefits to participants were that 'you benefit from national and international recognition of your Australian qualifications' which 'means that once you graduate you'll have the skills to meet the needs of your industry at home, in Australia or even further afield' (http://www.aptc.edu.au). Opening the programme in Fiji the Australian High Commissioner emphasized that graduates would be 'more competitive in domestic and global skilled labour markets'. A new skilled migration flow was imminent.

While nothing came of a possible regional nursing college, a series of changes in policy and practice demonstrate the contemporary shift to the deliberate export of semi-skilled workers, through programmes established in New Zealand and Australia, supported by island states. While SHWs are yet to be formally part of this, the shift towards interest in export rather than stability or return is evident. Hitherto such 'managed migration' in the Pacific has involved semi-skilled or unskilled workers, such as the phosphate miners and maritime workers of Kiribati and Tuvalu, and agricultural workers in New Zealand. In each case these were workers for whom domestic demand was weak, rather than being in areas of considerable national shortage where training costs are high. Significantly, at the same time that both the Caribbean and the Pacific regions have begun to contemplate and even organize formal labour export, there is growing evidence that the Philippines has almost literally 'sold out', since the outflow of workers is no longer an overspill but now affects the functioning of the health system, especially in regional areas (Connell 2008c). For small island states, where labour reservoirs are necessarily restricted by small size, this 'second generation' problem suggests an ominous precedent.

The shift outwards has occurred despite the evidence of exploitation of some unskilled Pacific island workers and doubts over the willingness of recipient countries to develop more ethical recruitment systems for skilled workers, especially SHWs, that would provide some basis for reciprocity and compensation. Metropolitan countries have found it easier, and much cheaper, to recruit SHWs from overseas, rather than train locally, partly because they are better and more quickly able to direct migrant workers to sectors or regions of shortage. Destination countries have consequently taken only some policy directions that would slow the migration of skilled workers. Following the precedent of a Commonwealth Code, in 2006 the independent Pacific island states developed a Pacific Code of Practice to regulate recruitment of SHWs. The Code focused on principles of transparency, fairness and mutuality of benefits, where, for example, 'recruiters should not seek to recruit health workers who have an outstanding obligation to their own country' (WHO and SPC 2006: 4). As the Code is voluntary, and there is limited direct recruitment of SHWs in the region, its impact may be slight, but its existence attests to existing migration problems and is effectively a residual attempt to staunch the flow.

A POLICY VACUUM?

In an ideal world the need for SHWs would be reduced by improved health, but that is as unlikely in the Pacific as anywhere else, and movement towards PHC remains an ideal. Indeed, the simultaneous transition towards NCDs and longer life expectancies has increased the need for SHWs, as it has elsewhere, and demanded larger budgets. Equally, there is little possibility of significant technological changes, such as telemedicine

(Smith 2004) or robotics, that might reduce demand. Nor has accelerated migration reduced demand since most migrants are young.

Despite widespread and long-standing recognition of the potential utility of particular policy directions and packages, limited implementation has resulted from a lack of finance to develop some programmes (better wages and technology), resistance (to nurse practitioners) and, above all, the lack of political will and management (some lost through migration) to implement and monitor programmes effectively. In-country education with a local curriculum reduces attrition and migration more effectively than overseas education, but its practice challenges the cultures of migration, and even the 'non-exportable' specialized master's degree at FScM proved all too transportable.

There are substantial gulfs between plans, especially when formulated by consultants, and reality. In the Marshall Islands the Strategic Development Plan had as its principal objective: 'Achieving an enhanced dynamic primary health care system to create greater awareness by empowering our people in order to motivate them to take initiatives in partnership to promote preventive healthy lifestyles' (Marshall Islands 2001a: 35). Yet 'the same patients come back to outpatients day after day, since they expect to be better the next day and do not understand that it takes time and they must maintain their medications'. However, 'in the wards we do not have time to teach, we do not even have time for a cup of coffee'. Strategies distanced from harsh reality were hard to implement, though one outcome has been a general pressure from aid donors for good governance and good 'housekeeping'.

Policies that might redress and reduce migration are implausible for small and poor island states, where the skill drain has been part of a wider migration stream that, for half a century, has provided real gains through human capital transfers (with return migration), so that remittances are the fastest growing elements of national economies. Regional intensification in the competition for SHWs has meant countries increasingly recruiting from each other, rather than addressing the 'more difficult' causes of attrition and shortage that are linked to inadequate wages and working conditions. Yet, without significant changes in national policy on both public health and migration in metropolitan recipient countries, attempts to slow the migration of SHWs must come from within the Pacific since they are unlikely to come from outside. In a world where public sector solutions go against the flow of contemporary history, stemming certain migration tides is a task of Canutian proportions, while state regulation is now more concerned with encouraging rather than preventing migration. Though there are at least two scales, policy intervention has very quickly moved away from specific interventions within the health sector, that might influence scholarships, wages and conditions of work etc., to more national perspectives that involve the managed migration of a significant proportion of the workforce. In the end the key solution is as simple and as challenging as ensuring that health receives a rather greater effective share of the national budget.

8 At the End of the Chain?

> Three decades ago the Samoan government's concern was over the fact that there was almost no Samoan with specialised skills. Training more people was seen to be the solution. Today, the worry is that as more people receive higher education more are also leaving the country. (Liki 1994: 144)

Accelerated emigration has helped to establish small and vulnerable Pacific island states as irrevocably a peripheral and dependent part of a wider world. Contemporary migration has expanded, diversified, become more skilled, more complex and with more dispersed destinations. Demographic structures have changed and shifted, as island states, individuals and international agencies have attached new and increased significance to migration, remittances and the role of the diaspora, in contexts where conventional development strategies, centred on agriculture or tourism, have achieved limited success. The life-courses of Pacific islanders, present or absent, increasingly involve international ties, as island states and their peoples have sought out new opportunities. Experiences and perceptions of the wider world, its values and its material rewards underlie the migratory experience and, in an electronic era where numerous relatives are overseas, knowledge of distant places is less fragmentary. Migration is now an appropriate and legitimate means to economic and social well-being, rather than a rupture or discontinuity with island experiences. Yet it has also become more selective, but also in greater demand at home and abroad, with part of that selectivity favouring women. Skilled Pacific health workers have become part of a global care chain from the Pacific islands to the metropolitan rim and beyond, to the UAE and the United Kingdom.

Small island states in some ways lend themselves to migration. Variants of blackbirding first introduced many islanders to a wider world. Small size, sometimes high population densities and governments where family and kinship relations are not unusual create a degree of intimacy, an absence of confidentiality and an intensity of social relationships. An occasional inability to separate personal and private life inhibits the ordinary performance of routine activities, stifles innovation and fails to reward merit.

Opportunities are necessarily limited, even with the best will in the world, in small-scale systems. Smallness and familiarity discourage cooperation as much as they encourage it, while scrutiny and conformity overwhelm individual desires for change. Social ties in island microstates are so powerful and pervasive that anonymity, impersonal role relationships and informality are difficult to maintain. When such systems are poorly financed, spread over many distant islands and short of human resources, management challenges are enormous and outcomes unsatisfactory. With limited opportunities, demanding working conditions and increased familiarity with other countries, migration has become an established option and a potential realization of household dreams: the outcome of a now established culture of migration where it is positive, acceptable and sometimes seemingly inevitable.

Migration occurs in a context where governments and institutions in developed countries have implemented recruitment campaigns to attract doctors and nurses, a situation evident by the 1960s and increasingly becoming global (Mejia, Pizurki and Royston 1979; Kingma 2006). Intensified global structures of demand, as developed countries face their own problems of recruitment, attrition and migration (for much the same reasons), ensure that relatively poor island states experience losses of SHWs and a declining ability to meet national health needs. Political fragility emphasizes such problems where skilled workers, well connected overseas, are relatively easily able to take flight. The rise of metropolitan demands coincided with stagnation of the economies of Pacific island states, many of which now exhibit high levels of unemployment and visible evidence of poverty. Tourism has kept several states afloat but economic growth has been less than in almost every other part of the world. Aid has sustained governments and remittances have sustained households. With limited budgets, small island states have been unable to restructure and modernise health care systems—or provide incomes and broader working conditions—comparable to those in developed countries. Uneven development is writ small, while the youth bulge, and the loss of safety nets reinforce the new outward urge.

EMBRACING A CULTURE OF MIGRATION

The establishment of a culture of migration, initially emerging in the small Polynesian states where migration was pervasive and set within historical precedents, and where decisions to migrate were part of everyday experiences and generally accepted as appropriate and legitimate means to economic and social well-being, transformed demography. If small states lent themselves to migration, so obtaining a skill emphasized the probability. Modernity, technology, interesting complications and the relief of boredom lie elsewhere. Skilled individuals, equally bound into social networks and extended families, were most likely to seek out new opportunities. A more technical culture of migration within the medical profession (but extending into other health arenas and some other skilled employment, such as aviation and sport) thus emphasized and enhanced the established socioeconomic culture of migration in further stressing what was absent in island contexts and what was necessary for 'proper' professional development.

Far beyond the Pacific there is a remarkable consensus and consistency over why SHWs migrate, centred on uneven development and hinging around wages and present and anticipated working conditions. Migration is primarily for economic reasons, a function of limited opportunities in island states, but embedded in a social context which emphasizes duty, service and reciprocity, resulting in sustained contacts across the diaspora and significant remittance flows. Such a rationale is broadly true both of small island states elsewhere (Connell and Conway 2000; Connell 2007e) and for other skilled workers (Voigt-Graf, Iredale and Khoo 2007). At the core of the parallel and similar problems of attrition and emigration are issues of management and human resource planning. Wages and poor working conditions are necessary yet insufficient causes for migration, since many SHWs (and other skilled workers) do stay in the region. Those who stay are often older or, conversely, recent graduates, with strong local family ties. Those who migrate have usually been working for a relatively short time (around four or five years—so often the bonding period), enough to gain experience and hone skills. Income is a major influence on decisions to join the health profession, for all SHWs, and a key influence on decisions to leave it or migrate. Migration demonstrates considerable sensitivity to income disparities, whether real or relative, regional or international. However, international migration also reflects dissatisfaction with the terms and conditions of government work, only part of which concerns income, emphasizing the institutional context of skilled migration.

Migrants stress extended family contexts, as education is directed towards income-generating opportunities where the rewards flow back home. In a sense, migration is embedded in the 'roots' of migrants' social relationships, and in the 'routes' taken to achieve success overseas. The notion of a 'transnational corporation of kin' is alluring in its combination of the extended family and strategic decision-making. While SHWs emphasize 'family strategies' that seek positive outcomes for children and parents in different continents, the quest for modernity, embodied in the 'two cultures' view of migration, indicates that self-interest and individual agency are also key elements, particularly for the migration of skilled workers. In this dual culture, migration is simultaneously expected, desired and also feared as families are fragmented (O'Meara 1990: 70); as has been observed in a parallel context 'the paradox of transnationalism is that families make strategic decisions to separate in order to maintain family unity and to advance the welfare of children' (Kobayashi and Preston 2007: 151). A moral economy is thus writ large. Not only is there both 'creative ambiguity and controlled paradox' (Chapman 1991: 290) but migration decisions are embedded in social structures where sometimes vague (but understandable) statements about income gains or seeking a 'better life' do not necessarily translate into western goals, insofar as these too can be pinned down.

Migration is invariably selective. The present focus on SHWs obscures the loss of other skilled groups, many in the public sector, such as IT workers, academics, teachers, airline pilots and a host of others, spilling over into a significant loss of sportsmen and tradesmen, less likely to be employed in the public service. Particular specialisms may be critically affected. In 2006 Fiji was experiencing a shortage of meteorologists, employing two expatriates to compensate as migration had taken its toll and scholarships were rarely forthcoming for such specialized positions. The Director of the Meteorology Department noted that 'the problem was rampant, not just in Fiji or in the region, as meteorologists tend to look for better opportunities elsewhere . . . those in Fiji normally migrate to Australia or New Zealand whereas weather forecasters there tend to look for opportunities in Canada and the United States' (*Fiji Times*, 4 July 2006). The Pacific was a small link in other global chains. Even Niue experiences a shortage of such jobs as car mechanics, electricians, carpenters and TV repairers, to the extent that the limited migration into Niue from the Philippines and other Pacific island states is mainly of tradesmen. Skills are increasingly in deficit. As migration has become more selective and more permanent, so the skill loss is more evidently a brain drain. Certainly destination countries are more anxious for skilled workers than for those once destined for the 'secondary sector' so necessary for the expanding manufacturing sectors of the 1970s. Despite the new guest worker schemes migration is widely seen to be for the skilled and denied to the unskilled. In Fiji, for example, the cost of inequitable national development policies is said to have:

> been borne by the very grassroots of society, Fijians as well as non-Fijians [Indo-Fijians] who have no skills or resources to escape to a greener pasture—an option the best and brightest of both communities have exercised . . . There is hardly any evidence of this magnitude of loss of human capital by any other society during peace times, and it is even harder to imagine that any society can remain viable if struck by such a calamity. (Shah 2007: 27)

In different ways Pacific islanders are caught up in a multitude of uneven global migration chains that have irrevocably changed the destinies of individuals, households and countries.

Distinctive in much of the Pacific is the manner in which small island populations have stabilized and declined as migration has intensified. In every Pacific island state outside Melanesia the population balance continues to shift gradually overseas, because of the presence of kin, education and employment opportunities there. While return migrants bring back skills, technological expertise and capital, there are all too few of them, especially in the public sector. Families with kin spread across countries have developed new transnational forms of family life, increasingly characterized by ambivalence to ancestral homes (Lee 2003, 2007). Island families have absorbed changes to local culture, and the social costs of disrupted extended households, because of the inexorable logic of migration and its economic benefits. In so doing, what was once a culture of mobility, or circulation, has become a culture of migration.

ISLANDERS IN THE GLOBAL HEALTH CARE CHAIN

Even in the 1930s health workers were brought from PNG for a very limited training in Australia, and by the 1940s Samoans were taking up nursing scholarships in New Zealand; many sophisticated skills have conventionally been taught in the metropolitan states. Islanders went home after training and it was not until the 1970s that both the loss of some trainees and the later migration of others began to represent an incipient and still localized brain drain (Bartsch 1974). By the 1980s, for Samoa at least, 'the departure of well-trained people has increased from a "brain-drain" to a dangerous torrent' (O'Meara 1990: 5). That was an understandable exaggeration, yet, by the 1990s, though the trickle had scarcely become a flood, except after Fijian coups, losses were more substantial and more widespread. In the same decade the migratory chains grew longer as SHWs moved to Dubai, South Africa, the United Kingdom, the United States and elsewhere. Pacific islanders had worked in many such places before but most were men and few were health workers. The slow feminization of the migrant Pacific island labour force, emphasized in SHW migration, would have been more pervasive were it not that most nurses are married women, and husbands provided or even demanded stability.

Conventionally the global care chain has been linked to the migration of women, as unskilled domestic workers, nannies and caregivers have been employed in general childcare and 'eldercare', where migrants are poorly paid, often exploited and beyond the reach of ethical principles, labour legislation and even kindness. A growing, but quite immeasurable, number of Pacific islanders have taken up such positions in each of the metropolitan states. Many such migrants are disadvantaged within metropolitan labour markets, and they and some SHWs have been deskilled during migration. Such outcomes, however disappointing, are for some superior to what has been left behind.

The care chains that involve SHWs extend beyond those of the unskilled and deskilled. From the 1970s onwards they took in the four metropolitan states, with New Zealand the greatest beneficiary of these voluntary and later recruited skilled labour streams. The United States gained least as SHWs found it harder to gain recognition there. By the end of the century the chains were more complex. Within the Pacific once wealthy Nauru was linked to independent states like Fiji, and regular flows from south of the equator went to the aid-dependent states of Palau and Marshall Islands. The last phase of complexity coincided with the onset of active recruiting in the region at the start of the twenty-first century and migration to UAE, Bermuda and the United Kingdom. This final phase, exclusively of nurses, and primarily of the most competent and highly trained (such as ICU nurses)—recruited as much by word of mouth as by advertisement—has marked the growing independence of women and the new status, prestige and economic rewards from such extended chains. Enhanced status has been a typical outcome of the international migration of female SHWs (Connell 2008c), alongside economic gains and some social costs.

While the Pacific is a relatively late entrant into the global care chain it is not at the end of that chain. As Pacific SHWs have been recruited and migrated elsewhere so island states have intensified their own overseas recruitment. Their financial status has condemned them to some frustration in seeking from the dwindling pool of potential migrants from other developing countries; they may lose the 'best and the brightest' but they rarely gain them. Many doctors have come from countries (such as Burma) that were beset with political problems, others in search of superior incomes and new experiences. Here, in its turn, the Pacific has gained at the expense of distant places, though that gain is slight in comparison with the extent of emigration. In an emerging world of hypermobility the best SHWs have a range of choices. The *Cook Islands Herald* recorded with some anguish in 2006 that a Saudi doctor (holding an Australian passport) had lasted just one week in the Cook Islands before returning to Australia but that even she had lasted longer than the doctor she 'replaced' who, whilst en route from Germany, had simply changed his mind and returned home (13 June 2006). Isolated Pacific island states are poorly placed to compete.

The costs of global mobility are unevenly borne by the poorer sending countries and the benefits are concentrated in recipient countries. These may also be intraregional as a two-tier system emerges: from poorer island states to richer ones, and from all of them to the metropoles. As yet there has been no compensation for this transfer, or perverse migration, of human resources, hence growing concern over the ethics involved in the migration of scarce SHWs from poorer countries where health problems are more substantial and pressing. The Pacific is simply part of a broader structure of the 'cherry-picking' (less elegantly 'poaching') of skilled workers amidst the greater selectivity of migration policies in developed countries, that have yet to resolve domestic human resource issues, within a current global deficit of some four million SHWs.

THE IMPACT OF LOSS: THE WORST OF TIMES?

There is a widespread belief that the impacts of SHW migration have worsened, with greater competition for workers and intensified recruitment, as migrant numbers increase and the care chain becomes global. However, health services have not been the recipients of steadily increasing resources either in relative or absolute terms; to improve services without additional resources requires a willingness to innovate, experiment and adapt, particularly difficult without committed staff. Distinguishing the impacts of migration and inadequate funding is impossible. However, the density of SHWs correlates closely with better health outcomes, least evident in Melanesia where densities are low and disease burdens are greatest. The impact of loss (including attrition), though still partly anecdotal, is evident in overwork, depleted morale and less adequate health care systems in most of the region, especially rural and remote areas, which are not compensated by return migration, replacement or remittances. As health consumers in rural areas make individual rational choices and move to urban areas for medical care so the collective ability to demand more effective regional services is reduced.

What occurs in the health sector also happens with other skilled workers though, arguably, teachers apart, few migrate from areas of such national importance. Moreover, the loss of SHWs from rural areas, and the lack of adequate education and health services in some remote islands, is just one example of the way in which Pacific island peripheries have been gradually marginalized. As populations move away, transport infrastructure decays and economic production withers, social and economic stagnation have followed. What might once have been a 'pampered periphery' in early post-colonial times is now a neglected and abandoned periphery. Smaller islands particularly, like Namoluk in Micronesia, have experienced a 'brain drain' as the brightest children moved away to high school, training and jobs elsewhere, teachers (and health workers) reluctantly moved to such islands, educational levels fell, islanders were less easily able to compete in the wider world (Marshall 2004: 69) and their islands were less attractive destinations for skilled workers. The sequel was further migration.

At a wider scale there are more than hints of the emergence of a downward spiral, where the loss of human capital and financial capital by emigration reduces the capacity of island economies, leading to fewer opportunities and further migration. The departure of even a few skilled workers has significant consequences, whether for nations or remote areas. Human resources are both valuable and fragile. 'With the manpower [sic] chain thinly stretched . . . a single break in it, through sickness, absence for training or emigration, can cause disruption and considerable loss of efficiency' (Shand 1980: 16). Both internal and international migration of SHWs exemplify and exacerbate urban bias and the 'inverse care law'.

The skill drain provides some gains to sending countries through human capital transfers (with return migration), remittances and the investments of returnees. Given the proliferation of transnational corporations of kin it would be disappointing if there were no household gains. Remittances compensate for skill losses, though they largely flow to the private sector and only incidentally support the public sector where most skills have been generated. Moreover, remittances are maintained for very long time periods, emphasizing that migrants are ultimately motivated by factors beyond altruistic family support, such as asset accumulation and investment at 'home', as the intergenerational flow of remittances takes on more individualistic elements (Brown 1998). Even so remittances epitomize a moral economy where affective ties and social norms ensure that as long as there are needy kin in the islands remittances will reach them. Such private gains only indirectly filter through to the public sector. The bulk of existing evidence points to overall economic losses in sending countries and gains to receiving countries, especially as migration has gradually shifted to respond to demand. What for health care is a perverse migration is a private gain for many households.

Return is minimal, other than after bonding. So many SHWs, many with partners with similar skills, can achieve a comfortable life in their destinations, which only a sense of duty—professional or personal—can disturb. When this study first began a Tongan public servant commented, not entirely in jest, that there was little point asking Tongans why they had chosen to return to the country because all would simply say 'for God, King and country'. A Fijian doctor in New Zealand said, 'We have lost our patriotism in Fiji. No one person or the Ministry can curb emigration. If there is a sense of belonging to the country, no salary, no attraction will be greater than to serve one's motherland. Many no longer feel that about this motherland, this birthright phenomenon' (quoted in Naidu 1997: 82). Even allowing for much hyperbole, and the absence of significant return migration, such statements are indicative of the very powerful attachment to 'home', the strong social ties that link islanders to home and the manner in which the structure of community, whatever that entails at various levels, may influence return migration. For most, however, remittances have taken the place of return.

A COLONIAL LEGACY?

Colonial health services were highly centralized, short of human and fiscal resources and often unable to service remote areas without mission support. After independence the primacy of central hospitals briefly declined, decentralization was promoted, and though training of adequate numbers of SHWs barely met national needs, a national service was tangible. Subsequent budgetary shortfalls, the reluctance of SHWs to work in remote locations, aid to central hospitals and migration have produced a health system that closely resembles its colonial predecessors, with many of the failures of outreach identified in the 1970s (Davidson 1980) again evident.

Pacific health systems are fragile and poorly funded with a continued bias towards more costly curative care services that are heavily reliant on SHWs. Low expenditure has meant that PHC is weak and several systems are characterized by a litany of disappointment: a shortage of SHWs (even before migration), weak middle management, poor information systems, inadequate policy and regulatory frameworks, unreliable supply of drugs and medical supplies (especially in remote areas) and outdated equipment and infrastructure. Public spending cuts have made management more difficult, but even more crucial, hence the widespread focus of aid donors on 'good governance'. Few island health plans have actively addressed human resource issues, while others have failed because of poor design, unrealistic goals, lack of local ownership and a simple failure to implement them (because of finance or poor management) in a context where 'health information systems have been described as the world's biggest information cemetery' (Kuartei 2005: 155). At a national level health care rarely has priority, resources is poorly aligned towards outcomes, accountability is lacking and few incentives support the effective delivery of services.

Island governments have not usually sought to intervene in the process of international migration, and are unlikely to do so in the future, because of the financial benefits and because decision-makers are potential migrants. The 'safety valve' effect, limited economic growth and concern over individual freedom of movement, have combined to result in steady and domestically unimpeded outmigration. The migration of SHWs is merely part of a wider migration stream and attempts to single them out for special policy intervention would be unlikely to succeed. In a context of stagnating economies and some degree of aid fatigue (and even the migration of middle managers), the context for policy intervention is being eroded. With limited resources health systems in the Pacific can never compare or compete with those in developed countries.

'Managed migration', seemingly attractive within the certainty of international migration, offers barely a Band-Aid. If there was no real overseas demand for health workers then migration might decline (especially to distant places), but it would not end, as people move for multiple reasons. However, developed countries, similarly engaged in processes of privatisation and restructuring, have not usually made working conditions in the public sector more favourable or produced enough local SHWs, while the arrival of the 'baby boom' generation at retirement has increased demand. Nonetheless, the onus has increasingly shifted towards the role of recipient countries in ensuring that, if migration is to continue, then it be more equitable and that there be compensation for losses incurred in sending countries. Thus far recipient countries have generally been either unable or unwilling to change a migration system that provides substantial benefits to them.

TOWARDS THE FUTURE: THE BEST OF TIMES?

While international migration has had both positive and negative effects in the Pacific, the significance of the positive effects (particularly increased standards of living) must be contrasted with the limited development potential of many states and their failure to achieve economic growth or sustainable development. Over a quarter of a century ago, the greater self-sufficiency that would have followed a decline of migration and remittances would have been difficult and painful (Connell 1981). Expectations never decline. Despite greater inequalities in sending societies, migration has provided new and welcome opportunities. Pragmatism has overwhelmed intellectual doubts; short-term need has triumphed over long-term planning. Demand for migration and remittances is likely to be sustained, alongside rising expectations, in conditions of limited national economic growth. The voices of those who urge more self-reliant development strategies have been stilled. A new diaspora has remarkably quickly come to characterize contemporary Pacific island states.

Outside Melanesia, as many islanders are overseas as at 'home', whilst in the smallest Polynesian states the balance has overwhelmingly shifted overseas. Notions of home thus change, provoking anxious and partisan debates over the extent to which cultures are retained or transformed, and become hybrid or syncretic, resulting in new phrases such as 'rooted cosmopolitanism' (Clifford 2001) to reflect the clash or combination of new residences, roots and routes. Traditions become reconstructed, articulated in ever changing forms and evident across now deterritorialized nations, islands and cultures. Whilst identities may be hybrid and hyphenated, they may also, as in the case of Samoans in New Zealand, represent successful cosmopolitans 'at ease in multiple worlds, rather than natives of place torn by new and multiple allegiances' (Yi-Fu Tuan, quoted in Western 1992: 269). While cultures shift, citizenship changes and new loyalties emerge, economic ties to home have remained remarkably resilient.

Migrants and their children remain 'migrants' though their identities have changed. New technology has made connectivity both more fashionable and more feasible, as the Pacific, fully a third of the earth's surface, has experienced a new 'cartography of compression' (Kempf 1999), where telephones, email and chat pages have created 'cyber-Polys' (Morton 1999). Home nations and islands remain powerful unifying symbols for migrants and their children. Hence, in these new transnational societies and:

> [i]n an uncertain global political economy, even the most cosmopolitan Samoan must ensure that Samoa is not merely a nostalgic fantasy, but a potentially real destination. . .. Migration is rarely absolute, unambivalent or final; it is not a cause and consequence of a definite break with a cultural life that is part of history, but a partial and conditional state, characterised by ambiguity and indeterminacy. A fixed status presupposes that the future can be foretold. Uncertainty defines the experience of migration, even in second generations. (Connell 1995: 277)

Contraction of the world through migration and electronics, and their consequences, from remittances to inter-regional kinship, have widened international ties yet, ultimately, have also ensured that symbolically and practically, especially through land tenure, islanders rarely abandon island homes. Indeed, as Marshall has phrased it, while 'people are no longer bound to places, they are still bound up in them' (2004: 145). Homelands will remain anchors and touchstones; geographical ties endure.

Migration has become an ever more conscious household strategy, because of its crucial role in generating remittances, so orienting education, training and employment to careers with scope for migration. In parallel with the individual and household embrace is the growing assumption throughout human resource planning in the region that some migration will ensue. A recent report on the standardization of nurse training in the Pacific quietly noted that all countries should be supported 'to enable an increase in the intakes in Schools of Nursing to prepare sufficient nurses to cover both local needs and anticipated nurse migration' (Usher et al. 2007: 7). It is not yet evident that states themselves are training SHWs for migration, but there are precedents in Kiribati and Tuvalu where seamen are trained for overseas labour markets. Australia has begun a training programme for Kiribati nursing students to provide them with international qualifications. There is slow movement towards a Pacific variant of the 'Philippines model' of training an excess of SHWs to join the 'global care chain'. The opening of the Australia-Pacific Technical College, ostensibly to strengthen island skills, but also 'to meet domestic demands and increase access to international labour markets' (Chapter 7), emphasizes the shift to a new selectivity, as a wider range of workers acquire international qualifications with the collaboration and direction of metropolitan states.

Policies are currently oriented towards increased rather than reduced migration: national goals are coalescing with household goals, as most states are seeking out migration options for skilled and unskilled workers alike. The narrow yet open economies of the region are increasingly influenced by transitions in the international economic system, and particularly the superior growth of Pacific Rim nations, that has enabled migration. The new outward urge is becoming consolidated, nationalized and institutionalized as a new, loosely self-inflicted neocolonialism emerges.

In this century alone there has been a spectacular increase in overseas migration from the Pacific, but also an unmet demand for it, from individuals whose dreams might turn to dust, and from governments, who have put increased pressure on countries such as Australia, to relax what are perceived to be overly restrictive and even unethical policies. After around thirty years of independence, and disappointment over the challenges and fruits of development, such interests and pressures are now spilling over into Melanesia. If Tonga was 'a society in centrifugal motion' (Marcus 1993: 32) over a decade ago, so the whole Pacific now fits that disposition. Migration, already changing fast, may be on the verge of taking quite new forms. While the Pacific will not become the 'earth's empty quarter' (Ward 1989), it will be increasingly dependent on migration opportunities elsewhere.

In a globalized world small island states in every ocean face uncertain times. Most island states have become increasingly similar to those in the more impoverished sub-Saharan African states where four factors (with the obvious change of land to sea)—a conflict trap, a natural resources trap (with its ensuing 'resource curse'), being landlocked with bad neighbours and bad governance in a small country—have held back development (Collier 2007). The rhetoric and rare practice of self-reliance, at national and household levels, have disguised a situation in which there has been a growing dependence on external sources of funding, whether from aid, remittances or investment, and a wide-ranging poverty of opportunities. While accelerated national and international migration has been partly a response to the collapse of commodity markets, the stagnation of tourism and the inability to effectively diversify domestic economies, it has nonetheless long been an effective strategy for economic diversification. The creation of new diasporas has spread economic risk beyond small nations and resulted in a considerable dependence on remittances, but has sheltered and protected small states in contexts where migration offers less risk than any outdated concentration on commodities. While migration may fracture families, albeit willingly, and contribute to new forms of socioeconomic inequality and incipient class formation (though ethnic and regional divisions and traditional power structures are of pervasive importance), engagement with the globalizing world through migration has become an acceptable and effective means of strengthening the resilience of fragile island households and economies.

At a very different scale, and from far away, international agencies, undoubtedly in a context of gathering aid fatigue, are increasingly stressing the role of diasporas in national development—an unreasonable focus on the potential role of emigrants, not least because their remittances support households rather than the nations they have moved away from. The social and emotional costs of such a new form of 'international self-reliance' are inherently problematic.

The international migration of SHWs has increased because perceptions of inadequate local conditions have grown, overseas 'host' populations have grown, demand has increased and recruitment intensified but, finally, because health skills are now valuable commodities in international migration. The shift from a more broadly based structure of migration towards more skilled migration has created a new dimension of inequality. No longer are the poor easily able to move (though that was never easy, at least from independent states) whereas the relatively rich (or at least those who have acquired training and marketable skills) are actively courted and recruited. There is growing international competition not just for 'the creative class' (Florida 2005) but for a wide range of skilled workers.

International migration has deferred and mitigated, but not resolved, broad development issues. The combination of weak economies, overburdened bureaucracies, urban unemployment, fractured social networks and uneven development challenge notions of sustainable development, the achievement of the MDGs and healthy islands. Small states are likely to remain weak for the foreseeable future, while becoming increasingly dependent on the wider world. International migration constitutes one increasingly less hesitant solution: a necessary bottom-up globalization that will always be both uneven and somewhat unsatisfying, as its resolution lies elsewhere. Yet it poses particular problems where island states are far from averse to the migration of unskilled and semi-skilled workers but unable to hold on to desperately needed skilled workers. It is nonetheless one means of linking into the benefits of globalization and a crucial means of building resilience by a specific spatial form of diversification. For the households of migrating SHWs it could be the best of times; for health services in small island states it may be the worst of times. Such ambiguities and uncertainties underpin migration. Little more than the ethical practices of so many health workers, for whom patients and professional service retain as much significance as personal and household aspirations, slow migration. For the moment, a sense of duty, family needs, pride, an ethic of service and simple inertia prevent the new global care chain overwhelming Pacific island states.

Bibliography

Abbott, D. (2007) Poverty and pro-poor policies for Pacific island countries. *Asia-Pacific Population Journal* 22 (3): 59–74.

Abbott, D. and S. Pollard. (2004) *Hardship and Poverty in the Pacific*. Manila: Asian Development Bank.

Adam, P. (2000) Experience and hopes for telehealth in Tokelau. *Pacific Health Dialog* 7 (2): 61–62.

Ahlburg, D. (1991) *Remittances and Their Impact: A Study of Tonga and Western Samoa*. Pacific Policy Papers No. 7. Canberra: ANU National Centre for Development Studies.

Ahlburg, D. and Levin, M (1990) *The North East Passage: A Study of Pacific Islander Migration to American Samoa and the United States*, Canberra: Australian National University National Centre for Development Studies Research Monograph No. 23.

Akl, E., N. Maroun, S. Major et al. (2007) Why are you draining your brain? Factors underlying decisions of graduating Lebanese medical students to migrate. *Social Science and Medicine* 64:1278–1284.

Anon. (2000) Samoan nurses nearly strike to achieve salary increase. *International Nursing Review* 47:134–136.

Asian Development Bank (ADB). (1996) *Tonga. Economic Performance and Selected Development Issues*. Manila: ADB.

———. (2000a) *Republic of the Fiji Islands. 1999 Economic Report*. Manila: ADB.

———. (2000b) *Samoa 2000*. Manila: ADB.

———. (2001) *Republic of the Marshall Islands. Meto 2000. Economic Report and Statement of Development Strategies*. Manila: ADB.

———. (2002a) *Tonga. Natural Resource Use and Sustainable Economic Development*. Manila: ADB.

———. (2002b) *Vanuatu. Economic Performance and Challenges Ahead*. Manila: ADB.

———. (2004) *Swimming Against The Tide. An Assessment of the Private Sector in the Pacific*. Manila: ADB.

———. (2005) *Towards a New Pacific Regionalism*. Manila: ADB.

———. (2006) *Juumemmej. Republic of the Marshall Islands Social and Economic Report 2005*. Manila: ADB.

Azam, A. (1996) *Motivation of Doctors within the Fiji Civil Service*. Unpublished MBA dissertation, University of the South Pacific, Suva.

Bailey, M., E. Khaiyum and V. Prasad. (2006) Fiji School of Medicine Diploma in Pharmacy graduates, ten year analysis—where are they now? *Pacific Health Dialog* 13 (2): 151–154.

Bakeea, M. (1991) Kiribati. In M. Bray (ed.), *Ministries of Education in Small States. Case Studies of Organisation and Management*, 247–264. London: Commonwealth Secretariat.

Baldacchino, G. (1997) *Global Tourism and Informal Labour Relations*. London: Mansell.

Ball, R. (1996) Nation building: the globalization of nursing—the case of the Philippines, *Pilipinas*, 27: 67–92.

Barclay, L., J. Fenwick, F. Nielson, B. Poston-Sanderson, P. Stowers and J. Wilkinson. (1998) *Samoan Nursing. The Story of Women Developing a Profession*. Sydney: Allen and Unwin.

Barker, J. (1994) Home alone: The effects of out-migration on Niuean elders' living arrangements and social supports. *Pacific Studies* 17:41–81.

Bartsch, W. (1973) *Higher Level Manpower in the South Pacific*. Suva: United Nations Development Advisory Team for the Pacific.

———. (1974) *The Skill Drain from Fiji. Situation and Possible Remedies*. Suva: Central Planning Office.

Bedford, R. , Mitchell, G. and Mitchell, M. (1980) Population History, in *Census of Niue 1976. Volume Two*, 4–19. Alofi: Government of Niue.

Bertram, G. (1986) Sustainable development in South Pacific micro-economies. *World Development* 14:809–822.

Bertram, I. and R. Watters. (1985) The MIRAB economy in South Pacific microstates. *Pacific Viewpoint* 26:497–520.

Boland, S. and B. Dollery. (2007) The economic significance of migration and remittances in Tuvalu. *Pacific Economic Bulletin* 22 (1): 102–114.

Booth, H. (1999) Pacific island suicide in comparative perspective. *Journal of Biosocial Science* 31:433–448.

Bouras, G. (1986) *A Foreign Wife*. Melbourne: Penguin.

Brown, M. (2000a) Flight of doctors deals body blows to the system. *Sydney Morning Herald*, 2 August.

———. (2000b) Yet another doctor gives up and packs his bags. *Sydney Morning Herald,* 3 August.

Brown, R. (1998) Do Pacific Island migrants' remittances decline over time? Evidence from Tongans and Western Samoans in Australia. *The Contemporary Pacific* 10:107–151.

Brown, R. and J. Connell. (2004) The migration of doctors and nurses from South Pacific Island nations. *Social Science and Medicine* 58:2193–2210.

———. (2006) Occupation-specific analysis of migration and remittance behaviour: Pacific island nurses in Australia and New Zealand. *Asia Pacific Viewpoint* 47:133–148.

Brunt, A. and C. Morris-Tafatu. (2002) *Review of NZODA Scholarships and Training in Niue*. Government of Niue.

Buchan, J. and F. O'May. (2000) Globalisation and healthcare labour markets: A case study from the United Kingdom. *Human Resources for Health Development Jouranal,* 4:111–118.

Bulicokocoko, A. (2002) *Industrial Issues for Nurses*. Unpublished paper presented to 10th South Pacific Nurses Forum, Brisbane, October.

Cama, T. and N. Smith. (2004) *Challenges and Actions for Nursing and Nurses in the South Pacific*. Unpublished paper presented to 12th South Pacific Nurses Forum, Rarotonga.

Chambers, A. and K. Chambers. (2001) *Unity of Heart. Culture and Change in a Polynesian Atoll Society*. Prospect Heights: Waveland Press.

Chand, S. (2007) Swim or sink: the predicament of the Fiji economy. *Pacific Economic Bulletin* 22 (2): 1–21.

Chapman, M. (1991) Pacific island movement and socioeconomic change: Metaphors of misunderstanding. *Population and Development Review* 17:263–292.

Chory-Assad, R. and R. Tamborini. (2001) Television doctors: An analysis of physicians in fictional and non-fictional television programs. *Journal of Broadcasting and Electronic Media* 45:499–521.

Christensen, P.M. (1995) *Infant Nutrition and Child Health on Tarawa, Kiribati.* University of New South Wales Pacific Studies Monograph No. 15, Sydney.

Clifford, J. (2001) Indigenous articulations. *The Contemporary Pacific* 13:468–490.

Cohen, J. (2004) *The Culture of Migration in Southern Mexico.* Austin: University of Texas Press.

Cohn, P. (2003) *Economic Independence through Expansion of Private Sector Enterprise—The 'Prescriptive Unreality' of Niue's Development Planning.* Working Paper No. 11, Melbourne University Private School of Development Studies.

Collier, P. (2007) *The Bottom Billion.* Oxford: Oxford University Press.

Commonwealth Secretariat. (2001) *Migration of Health Workers from Commonwealth Countries.* London: Commonwealth Secretariat.

Connell, J. (1981) Migration, remittances and rural development in the South Pacific. In G. Jones and H. Richter (eds.), *Population Mobility and Development: South East Asia and the Pacific*, 229–255. Canberra: ANU Development Studies Centre.

———. (1983) *Migration, Employment and Development in the South Pacific. Country Report No. 11. Niue.* Noumea: South Pacific Commission and International Labour Organisation.

———. (1987a) Migration, rural development and policy formation in the South Pacific. *Journal of Rural Studies* 3:105–121.

———. (1987b) Population growth and emigration: Maintaining a balance. In M. Taylor (ed.), *Fiji: Future Imperfect?*, 14–32. Sydney: Allen and Unwin.

———. (1989) Migrations, urbanisation et santé dans le Pacifique Sud. *Les Cahiers d'Outre Mer* 42:397–423.

———. (1995) In Samoan worlds. Culture, migration, identity and Albert Wendt. In R. King, J. Connell and P. White (eds.), *Writing Across Worlds. Literature and Migration*, 263–279. London: Routledge.

———. (1997) Health in Papua New Guinea: a decline in development. *Australian Geographical Studies* 35:271–293.

———. (2003a) Island dreaming: The contemplation of Polynesian paradise. *Journal of Historical Geography* 29:554–582.

———. (2003b) Losing ground? Tuvalu, the greenhouse effect and the garbage can. *Asia Pacific Viewpoint* 44:89–107.

———. (2003c) Regulation of space in the contemporary postcolonial Pacific city: Port Moresby and Suva. *Asia Pacific Viewpoint* 44:243–258.

———. (2005) A nation in decline? Migration and emigration from the Cook Islands. *Asian and Pacific Migration Journal* 14:327–350.

———. (2006a) Migration, dependency and inequality in the Pacific: Old wine in bigger bottles? In S. Firth (ed.), *Globalisation and Governance in the Pacific Islands*, 59–106. Canberra: Pandanus.

———. (2006b) Nauru: The first Pacific failed state. *The Round Table* 95:47–64.

———. (2006c) 'Saving the Solomons': A new geopolitics in the 'arc of instability'. *Geographical Research* 44:111–122.

———. (2007a) At the end of the world. Holding on to health workers in Niue. *Asian and Pacific Migration Journal* 16:179–198.

———. (2007b) 'The best island on the globe'. Constantly constructing tourism in Niue. *Australian Geographer* 38:1–13.

———. (2007c) The *Fiji Times* and the good citizen: Constructing modernity and nationhood in Fiji. *The Contemporary Pacific* 19:85–110.

———. (2007d) Islands, idylls and the detours of development. *Singapore Journal of Tropical Geography* 28:116–135.

———. (2007e) Local skills and global markets? The migration of health workers from Caribbean and Pacific island states. *Social and Economic Studies* 56:67–95.

———. (2008a) 'I never wanted to come home'. Skilled health workers in the South Pacific. In H. Lee and S. Francis (eds.), *Transnationalism and the Pacific Islands.* Canberra: ANU E Press.

———. (2008b) Niue: Embracing a culture of migration. *Journal of Ethnic and Migration Studies* 34: 1021–1040.

———. (2008c) Towards a global health care system. In J. Connell (ed.), *The International Migration of Health Workers*, 1–29. New York and London: Routledge.

———. (2009) 'We are so small'. Colonialism or autonomy in Tokelau. In G. Baldacchino and D. Milne (eds.), *The Case for Non-Sovereignty: Lessons from Sub-National Island Jurisdictions.* 161–173. London: Routledge.

Connell, J. and R. Brown. (2004) The remittances of migrant Samoan and Tongan nurses. *Human Resources for Health* 2 (2): 1–21.

———. (2005) *Remittances in the Pacific. An Overview.* Manila: ADB.

Connell, J. and D. Conway. (2000) Migration and remittances in island microstates: A comparative perspective on the South Pacific and the Caribbean. *International Journal of Urban and Regional Research* 24:52–78.

Connell, J. and R. King. (1999) Island migration in a changing world. In J. Connell and R. King (eds.), *Small Worlds, Global Lives: Islands and Migration*, 1–26. London: Pinter.

Connell, J. and J. Lea. (2002) *Urbanisation in the Island Pacific.* London: Routledge.

Connell, J. and B. Stilwell. (2006) Merchants of medical care: Recruiting agencies in the global health care chain. In C. Kuptsch (ed.), *Merchants of Labour*, 239–253. Geneva: ILO.

Connell, J. and C. Voigt-Graf. (2006) Towards autonomy? Gendered migration in Pacific island countries. In K. Ferro and M. Wallner (eds.), *Migration Happens. Reasons, Effects and Opportunities of Migration in the South Pacific*, 43–62. Vienna: Lit Verlag.

Connell, J., P. Zurn, M. Awases, B. Stilwell and J.M. Braichet. (2007) Sub-Saharan Africa: Beyond the health worker migration crisis? *Social Science and Medicine* 64:1876–1891.

Cowling, W. (1990) Motivations for contemporary Tongan migration. In P. Herda, J. Terrell and N. Gunson (eds.), *Tongan Culture and History,* 187–205. Canberra: Australian National University.

Coyne, T. (2000) *Lifestyle Diseases in Pacific Communities.* Noumea: Secretariat of the Pacific Community.

Crocombe, R. (1978) Rural development. *Pacific Perspective* 7 (1–2): 42–59.

Danser, S. (2005) *The Myths of Reality.* Loughborough: Heart of Albion Press.

D'Arcy, P. (2006) *The People of the Sea. Environment, Identity and History in Oceania.* Honolulu: University of Hawai'i Press

Davidson, L. (1980) Report on a visit to study health care delivery in a number of western Pacific islands. In Commonwealth Secretariat (ed.), *Special Health Problems of Island Developing and other Specially Disadvantaged Countries*, 79–92. London: Commonwealth Secretariat.

Davies, A. (1985) Small country blues. *Meanjin* 44:243–252.

Denoon, D. (1989) *Public Health in Papua New Guinea: Medical Possibility and Social Constraint, 1884–1984*. Cambridge: Cambridge University Press.
Dever, G. and S. Finau. (1995) The Yanuca Island declaration. *Pacific Health Dialog* 2 (2): 70–74.
Dewdney, J. (2000) *Kingdom of Tonga National Health Workforce Plan 2001–2020*. Nuku'alofa: Ministry of Health.
Dore, R. (1976) *The Diploma Disease*. London: Allen and Unwin.
Duncan, R. (2005) *Benefit-Cost Analysis of a Pacific Regional Nurse Training Facility* (mimeo). Suva: USP.
Durutalo, A. (2007) Fiji. *The Contemporary Pacific* 19:578–582.
Dusevic, T. (2001) Outwardly mobile. *Time*, 20–27 August: 30–33.
Easthope, H. (2002) *Migration, Education and Health in Kiribati. Understanding the Shortage of Skilled Health Professionals*. Unpublished BA (honours) thesis, University of Sydney.
Evans, M., R. Sinclair, C. Fusimalohi and V. Liava'a. (2002) Diet, health and the nutrition transition: Some impacts of economic and socio-economic factors on food consumption patterns in the Kingdom of Tonga. *Pacific Health Dialog* 9:309–315.
Faist, T. (2008) Migrants as transnational development agents: An inquiry into the newest round of the migration–development nexus. *Population, Space and Place* 14:21–42.
Fatupaito, M. (1997) American delinquents rehabilitated in Paradise—the inside story, *Talamua*, 4(1), February: 19–21.
Finau, S. (1988) Bureaucracy and the Pacific health services. *Journal of Pacific Studies* 14:131–144.
Finau, S., I. Wainoqolo and G. Cuboni. (2004) Health transition and globalization in the Pacific: Vestiges of colonialism? *Perspectives on Global Development and Technology* 3:109–129.
Firth, S. (1997) Colonial administration and the invention of the native. In D. Denoon (ed.), *The Cambridge History of the Pacific Islanders*, 253–288. Cambridge: Cambridge University Press.
Fisi'iahi, F. (2001) Labour migration from Tonga—of more benefit than harm? In V. Naidu, E. Vasta and C. Hawksley (eds.), *Current Trends in South Pacific Migration*, 41–53. Working Paper No. 7. Wollongong: Asia Pacific Migration Research Network.
Florida, R. (2005) *The Flight of the Creative Class. The New Global Competition for Talent*. New York: Harper.
Fong, M. (2003) *A Review of Options for Achieving an Adequate and Cost-Effective Supply of Appropriately Qualified Nurses for the Fijian Health System*. Unpublished paper presented to WHO Meeting on Migration of Skilled Health Personnel in Pacific Island Countries, Nadi.
Fusitu'a, P. (2000) *My Island Homes: Tonga, Migration and Identity*. Unpublished BA (honours) thesis, University of Sydney.
Gailey, C.W. (1992) State formation, development and social change in Tonga. In A. Robillard (ed.), *Social Change in the Pacific Islands*, 322–345, 464–5. London: Kegan Paul International.
Gani, A. (1999) Some dimensions of Fiji's recent emigration, *Pacific Economic Bulletin*, 15(1): 94–103.
Gee, T. (1970) *Manpower Planning—An Administrator's View*. Unpublished paper presented to South Pacific Seminar on Manpower Planning in the South Pacific, Suva.
Gewertz, D. and F. Errington. (1999) *Emerging Class in Papua New Guinea. The Telling of Difference*. Cambridge: Cambridge University Press.

———. (2007) The alimentary forms of the global life. *American Anthropologist* 109:496–508.
Gish, O. (1971) *Doctor Migration and World Health: The Impact of the International Demand for Doctors on Health Services in Developing Countries.* London: Bell.
Gish, O. and M. Godfrey. (1979) A reappraisal of the 'brain drain' with special reference to the medical profession. *Social Science and Medicine* 13:1–11.
Government of Kiribati. (1999) *Fourth Kiribati National Health Plan 1999–2002.* Tarawa: Ministry of Health.
Grieco, E. (2003) *The Remittance Behavior of Immigrant Households: Micronesians in Hawaii and Guam.* New York: LFB Scholarly Publishing LLC.
Hagopian, A., A. Ofusu, A. Fatusi, R. Biritwum, A. Essel, L. Hart et al. (2005) The flight of physicians from West Africa: Views of African physicians and their implications for policy. *Social Science and Medicine* 61:1750–1760.
Hammond, J. and J. Connell. (2009) The new blackbirds? Guestworker migration from Vanuatu to New Zealand. *New Zealand Geographer.* 65.
Hamnett, M. and J. Connell. (1981) Diagnosis and cure: The resort to traditional and modern medical practitioners in the North Solomons. *Social Science and Medicine* 15B:489–498.
Han, S. (1996) New horizons in health: A perspective for the 21st century. *Pacific Health Dialog* 2 (1): 253–258.
Hardill, I. and S. MacDonald. (2000) Skilled international migration: The experience of nurses in the United Kingdom. *Regional Studies* 34:681–692.
Harkness, L. (2001) Recent economic developments in the Kingdom of Tonga, *Pacific Economic Bulletin,* 16 (1): 19–43.
Hassall and Associates International. (1999) *Vanuatu Health Sector Planning and Management Development Report.* Canberra.
Hau'ofa, E. (1993) Our sea of islands. In E. Waddell, V. Naidu and E. Hau'ofa (eds.), *A New Oceania. Rediscovering Our Sea of Islands*, 2–16. Suva: University of the South Pacific.
Hayes, G. (1983) *Population of the Cook Islands.* Bangkok: ESCAP.
Hedson, J. (2000) Teleconsultations in Pohnpei State, Federated States of Micronesia. *Pacific Health Dialog* 7 (2): 46–50.
Henckel, T. (2006) Vanuatu's economy: Is the glass half empty or half full? *Pacific Economic Bulletin* 21 (3): 1–20.
Hess, J., K. Nero and M. Burton. (2001) Creating options: Forming a Marshallese community in Orange County, California. *The Contemporary Pacific* 13:89–121.
Heyn, J. (2003) *Migration and Development in Niue Island.* Unpublished MSc thesis, University of Montana, Missoula.
Hezel, F. (1989) Suicide and the Micronesian family. *The Contemporary Pacific* 1:43–74.
———. (2008) What's happened to all our college graduates? *Micronesian Counselor* 71.
Hezel, F. and M. Levin. (1996) New trends in Micronesian migration: FSM migration to Guam and the Marianas. *Pacific Studies* 19:91–114.
Hezel, F. and C. Lightfoot. (2005) Myths of the FSM economy. *Micronesian Counselor* 59.
Hirshman, J. (1980) Designing appropriate health delivery systems for the islands of the Pacific and Indian Oceans. In R. Shand (ed.), *The Island States of the Pacific and Indian Oceans*, 335–346. Canberra: ANU Development Studies Centre Monograph No. 23.
Hoadley, S. (1980) Aid, politics and hospitals in Western Samoa. *World Development* 8:443–455.

Hodge, A., G. Dowse, P. Toelupe, V. Collins et al. (1994) Dramatic increase in the prevalence of obesity in Western Samoa over the thirteen year period of 1978–1991. *International Journal of Obesity* 18:419–428.

Hooker, K. and J. Varcoe. (1999) Migration and the Cook Islands. In J. Overton and R. Scheyvens (eds.), *Strategies for Sustainable Development. Experiences from the Pacific*, 91–99. Sydney: UNSW Press.

Jacobs, B. (1975) Administrative problems of small countries. In P. Selwyn (ed.), *Development Policy in Small Countries*, 134–143. London: Croom Helm.

James, K. (1991) Migration and remittances: A Tongan village perspective. *Pacific Viewpoint* 32:1–23.

———. (2003) Is there a Tongan middle class? Hierarchy and protest in contemporary Tonga. *The Contemporary Pacific* 15:309–336.

Jenkins, M. and C. McSwain. (2005) The Republic of the Marshall Islands. In A. Marsella, A. Austin and B. Grant (eds.), *Social Change and Psychosocial Adaptation in the Pacific Islands,* 187–209. New York: Springer.

Kandel, W. and D. Massey. (2002) The culture of Mexican migration: A theoretical and empirical analysis. *Social Forces* 80:981–1004.

Kempf, W. (1999) Cosmologies, cities and cultural constructions of space: Oceanic enlargements of the world. *Pacific Studies* 22:97–114.

Ken, C. (2007) What's Killing Our Islanders? *Islands Business* 33 (3) March: 16–17.

———. (2008) Training islanders a top priority. *Islands Business* 34 (3): 42–43.

Kerslake, M. (1993) *The Nurse Practitioner in the South Pacific Region.* Unpublished MSc (PHC) thesis, Flinders University, Adelaide.

Kienene, T. (1993) Health care. In H. van Trease (ed.), *Atoll Politics. The Republic of Kiribati*, 250–257. Suva: Institute of Pacific Studies, USP.

Kingma, M. (2006) *Nurses on the Move. Migration and the Global Health Care Economy.* Ithaca, Cornell University Press.

Knapman, B. (1976) Indigenous involvement in the cash economy of Lau, Fiji, 1840–1946. *Journal of Pacific History* 11:167–188.

Kobayashi, A. and V. Preston. (2007) Transnationalism through the life course: Hong Kong immigrants in Canada. *Asia Pacific Viewpoint* 48:151–167.

Koloto, A. (2003) *National Survey of Pacific Nurses and Nursing Students.* Auckland: Loloto and Associates.

Koser, K. and J. Salt. (1997) The geography of highly skilled international migration. *International Journal of Population Geography* 3:285–303.

Kuartei, S. (2005) Health care plans and dust collection in the Pacific. *Pacific Health Dialog* 12 (2): 155–158.

Kupu, S. (2000) Health and telecast: A milestone for Tonga in the 21st century. *Pacific Health Dialog* 7 (2): 54–56.

Kuschel, R., A. Takiika and A. Kiu. (2005) Alcohol and drug use in Honiara, Solomon Islands. A cause for concern. In A. Marsella, A. Austin and B. Grant (eds.), *Social Change and Psychosocial Adaptation in the Pacific Islands,* 211–254. New York: Springer.

KVA Consult. (2007) Samoa economic update 2007. *Pacific Economic Bulletin* 22 (3): 1–14.

Laban, W. (2003) Speech to Samoan Nurses Association Conference. www.winnie.org.nz/speeches.

Lambert, S. (1941) *Doctor in Paradise.* Melbourne: Dent.

Lander, H. and V. Miles. (1992) *The Fiji School of Medicine, Pacific Studies Monograph No.* 2. Sydney: UNSW Centre for South Pacific Studies.

Leckie, J. (2000) Gender and work in Fiji: Constraints to re-negotiation. In A. Jones, P. Herda and T. Suaalii (eds.), *Bitter Sweet. Indigenous Women in the Pacific*, 73–92. Dunedin: University of Otago Press.

Lee, H. (2003) *Tongans Overseas. Between Two Shores*. Honolulu: University of Hawai'i Press.
———. (2004) All Tongans are connected: Tongan transnationalism. In V. Lockwood (ed.), *Globalization and Culture Change in the Pacific Islands*, 133–148. New Jersey: Pearson.
———. (2007) Transforming transnationalism: Second generation Tongans overseas. *Asian and Pacific Migration Journal* 16:157–178.
Leweniqila, M., L. Camaivuna and F. Dokoni. (2000) *Why are the Nightingales Flying Away?* (mimeo). Suva: Fiji Nurses Association.
Lewis, N. (1990) More than health services: Health for Pacific peoples. *Regional Development Dialogue* 11 (4): 76–96.
Lewis, N. and M. Rapaport. (1995) In a sea of change: Health transitions in the Pacific. *Health and Place* 1:211–226.
Liki, A. (1994) *E Tele A'A O Le Tagata. Career Choices of Samoan Professionals within and beyond their Nu'u Moni*. Unpublished MA thesis, University of the South Pacific, Suva.
———. (2001) Moving and rootedness: The paradox of the brain drain among Samoan professionals. *Asia-Pacific Population Journal* 16:67–84.
Lutua, K. (2002) *Salaries and Conditions of Employment for Nurses, Nurse Practitioners and Midwives—A Fijian Perspective*. Unpublished paper presented to 11th South Pacific Nurses Forum, Vila, August.
Macdonald, B. (1982) *Cinderellas of the Empire. Towards a History of Kiribati and Tuvalu*. Canberra: ANU Press.
McGrath, B. (1999) Swimming from island to island: Healing practice in Tonga. *Medical Anthropology Quarterly* 13:483–505.
Maclellan, N. (2007) Fiji, Iraq and Pacific Island security. *Race and Class* 48:47–62.
McMurray, C. (2004) Globalization and health: The paradox of the periphery. *Perspectives on Global Development and Technology* 3:91–108.
Macpherson, C. (1985) Public and private views of home: Will Western Samoan migrants return? *Pacific Viewpoint* 26:242–262.
———. (1992) Economic and political restructuring and the sustainability of migrant remittances: The case of Western Samoa. *The Contemporary Pacific* 4:109–136.
———. (1994) Changing patterns of commitment to island homelands: A case study of Western Samoa. *Pacific Studies* 17:83–116.
———. (2004) Transnationalism and transformation in Samoan society. In V. Lockwood (ed.), *Globalization and Culture Change in the Pacific Islands*, 165–181. New Jersey: Pearson.
Macpherson, C. and L. Macpherson. (1987) Toward an explanation of recent trends in suicide in Western Samoa. *Man* 22:305–330.
McPhetres, S. (2008) Commonwealth of the Northern Mariana Islands. *The Contemporary Pacific* 20:204–209.
Maddocks, I. (1975) Medicine and colonialism. *Australian and New Zealand Journal of Sociology* 11 (3): 27–33.
Manning, O. (1970) *Planning for Nursing Manpower in the South Pacific*. Unpublished paper presented to South Pacific Seminar on Manpower Planning in the South Pacific, Suva.
Marcus, G. (1981) Power on the extreme periphery: The perspective of Tongan elites in the modern world system. *Pacific Viewpoint* 22:48–64.
———. (1993) Tonga's contemporary globalizing strategies: Trading on sovereignty amidst international migration. In V. Lockwood, T. Harding and B. Wallace (eds.), *Contemporary Pacific Societies*, 21–33. Englewood Cliffs: Prentice Hall.

Maron, N. (2001) *Return to Nukunuku. Identity, Culture and Return Migration and Change to Tonga*. Unpublished BA (honours) thesis, University of Sydney.
Maron, N. and J. Connell. (2008) Return to Nukunuku. Employment, identity and return migration in Tonga. *Asia Pacific Viewpoint* 49: 168–184.
Marsh, K. (2007) Guam. *The Contemporary Pacific* 19:182–189.
Marshall, M. (2004) *Namoluk Beyond the Reef. The Transformation of a Micronesian Community*. Boulder: Westview.
Marshall Islands. (2001a) *Republic of the Marshall Islands. Strategic Development Plan Framework (2003–2018)*. Majuro: SEDP, Ministry of Finance.
Marshall Islands. (2001b) *Task Force Report. Majuro New Hospital*. Majuro: Ministry of Health and Environment.
Massey, D., Arango, J., Hugo, G., Kouaouci, A., Pellegrino, A. and Taylor, J. (1998) *Worlds in Motion*, New York: Oxford University Press.
Maude, H. (1981) *Slavers in Paradise*. Canberra: Australian National University Press.
May, R. and S. Tupouniua. (1980) The politics of small island states. In R. Shand (ed.), *The Island States of the Pacific and Indian Oceans*, 419–437. Canberra: ANU Development Studies Centre Monograph No. 23.
Mejia, A., H. Pizurki and E. Royston. (1979) *Physician Migration and Nurse Migration. Analysis and Policy Implications*. Geneva: WHO.
Miho, D. (2007) Palau. Nursing a system back to health. *Pacific* 32 (5) September–October: 45.
Mitchell, J. (2000) Violence as continuity: Violence as rupture. Narratives from an urban settlement in Vanuatu. In S. Dinnen and A. Ley (eds.), *Reflections on Violence in Melanesia*, 189–208. Sydney: Hawkins Press.
Mitchell, R. (1988) Fiji's health system since the coup. In S. Prasad (ed.), *Coup and Crisis: Fiji—A Year Later*, 75–78. Melbourne: Arena.
Mohanty, M. and V. Naidu. (2005) International migration, human capital loss and development in the South Pacific: The case of Fiji. In K. Ferro and M. Wallner (eds.), *Migration Happens. Reasons, Effects and Opportunities of Migration in the South Pacific*, 151–165. Vienna: Lit Verlag.
Morton, H. (1999) Islanders in space: Tongans online. In R. King and J. Connell (eds.), *Small Worlds, Global Lives: Islands and Migration*, 235–254. London: Pinter.
Muliaina, T. (2001) Remittances, the social system and development in Samoa. In V. Naidu, E. Vasta and C. Hawksley (eds.), *Current Trends in South Pacific Migration,* Working Paper No. 7, 20–40. Wollongong: Asia Pacific Migration Research Network.
Munro, D. and R. Bedford. (1980) Historical backgrounds. In *A Report on the Results of the Census of Tuvalu 1979*, 1–13. Funafuti, Government of Tuvalu.
Naidu, L. (1997) *Contemporary Professional Emigration from Fiji*. Unpublished MA thesis, University of the South Pacific, Suva.
Narayan, P. and R. Smyth. (2003) The determinants of emigration from Fiji to New Zealand. *International Migration* 41:33–58.
Newell, K. (1983) Primary health care in the Pacific. *Social Science and Medicine* 17:1441–1447.
Nietschmann, B. (1979) Ecological change, inflation and migration in the far western Caribbean. *Geographical Review* 69:1–24.
Nurse, K. (2004) Migration and development in the Caribbean. *Focal Point* (March): 3–5.
Oman, K. (2007) *Should I Migrate or Should I Remain? Professional Satisfaction and Career Decisions of Doctors who have Undertaken Specialist Training in Fiji*. Unpublished PhD thesis, James Cook University, Townsville.
Oman, K., S. Bale, W. Baravilala, J. Malani, E. McCaig, E. Rodgers and R. Moulds. (2006) Donor countries may unintentionally become major beneficiaries of their

own aid: The case of postgraduate specialist training at the Fiji School of Medicine. *Fiji Medical Journal* 27 (2): 11–18.

O'Meara, T. (1990) *Samoan Planters. Tradition and Economic Development in Polynesia*. Fort Worth: Holt Rinehart and Winston.

Oommen, T. (1989) India: 'Brain drain' or migration of talent? *International Migration* 27:411–422.

Ospina, H. (2006) Cuba exports health. *Le Monde Diplomatique* (August), 10.

Oulton, J. (1998) International trade and the nursing profession. In S. Zarrilli and C. Kinnon (eds.), *International Trade in Health Services: A Development Perspective*, 125–133. Geneva: UNCTAD and WHO.

Pak, S. and C. Tukuitonga. (2006) *Towards Brain Circulation: Building the Health Workforce Capacity in the Pacific Region*. Wellington: NZAID.

Pareti, S. (2007) Big ain't bad. *Islands Business* 33 (3) March: 21.

Parker, I. (2006) Birth of a nation? *The New Yorker*, 1 May: 66–75.

Petersen, G. (1979) External politics, internal economics and Ponapean social formation. *American Ethnologist* 6:25–40.

Pierantozzi, S. (2000) Palauans and guest workers: An opinion paper. *The Contemporary Pacific* 12:349–358.

Plant, C. (1977) The development dilemma. In C. Plant (ed.), *Rotuma. Split Island*, 173–189. Suva: Institute of Pacific Studies.

Poirine, B. (1997) A theory of remittances as an implicit family loan agreement. *World Development* 25:589–611.

Pollock, N. and S. Finau. (1999) Health. In M. Rapaport (ed.), *The Pacific Islands. Environment and Society*, 282–295. Honolulu: Bess Press.

Rafai, E. (2006) An outbreak of measles, Koro Island, 1997. *Pacific Health Dialog* 13 (2): 25–30.

Raghuram, P. and E. Kofman. (2002) The state, skilled labour markets and immigration: The case of doctors in England. *Environment and Planning A* 34:2071–2089.

Rallu, J.L. (1997) *Population, Migration, Développement dans le Pacifique Sud*. Paris: UNESCO.

Ramo, W. (1991) Solomon Islands. In M. Bray (ed.), *Ministries of Education in Small States*, 265–283. London: Commonwealth Secretariat.

Rees, T.P. (2000) Nurses show true meaning of sacrifice. *Samoa Observer*, 27 April.

Robertson, R. (2006) Fiji futuring: Connectivity and development. *Pacific Economic Bulletin* 21:22–35.

Rokoduru, A. (2008) Transient greener pastures in managed temporary labour migration: Fiji nurses in the Marshall Islands. In J. Connell (ed.), *The International Migration of Health Workers*, 171–180. New York and London: Routledge.

Rotem, A. (2007) *Addressing Challenges in Human Resource Development: Experience from a Pacific Island Nation*. Unpublished paper presented to International Symposium on Health Workforce, Lisbon (mimeo).

Rotem, A. and M. Bailey. (1999) *Health Personnel Migration within Commonwealth Countries in the Pacific Region* (mimeo). Sydney: UNSW.

Rotem, A. and J. Dewdney. (1991) *The Health Workforce. South Pacific Island Nations*. Sydney: WHO/UNSW.

Rubinstein, D. (1992) Suicide in Micronesia and Samoa: A critique of explanations. *Pacific Studies* 15:51–75.

———. (1999) Staking ground: Medical anthropology, health and medical services in Micronesia. In R. Kiste and M. Marshall (eds.), *American Anthropology in Micronesia*, 327–359. Honolulu: University of Hawai'i Press.

SAGRIC International. (2000) *A Review of the Health Sector in the Cook Islands.* Rarotonga: Ministry of Health, Government of the Cook Islands.
Samoa. (2000) *Samoa Nurses Association Country Report.* Unpublished paper presented to 10th South Pacific Nurses Forum, Brisbane, October.
Schoeffel, P. (1984) Dilemmas of modernization in primary health care in Western Samoa. *Social Science and Medicine* 19:209–216.
Schutz, B. and R. Tenten. (1979) Adjustment, problems of growth and change. In A. Talu (ed.), *Kiribati. Aspects of History*, 106–127. Suva: Institute of Pacific Studies.
Scott, G. (2003) Situating Fijian transmigrants: Towards racialised transnational social spaces of the undocumented. *International Journal of Population Geography* 9:181–198.
Secretariat of the Pacific Community. (2007) *Pacific Island Populations.* Noumea: SPC.
Seniloti, K. (2005) 'They are digging their graves with their teeth'. Mortality, poverty and nutrition in the Pacific. *Journal of Pacific Studies* 28:163–191.
Shah, S. (2007) When race sits at the root of all our problems. *Fiji Times*, 17 November: 26–27.
Shand, R. (1980) Island smallness: some definitions and implications. In R. Shand (ed.), *The Island States of the Pacific and Indian Oceans*, 3–20. Canberra: ANU Development Studies Centre Monograph No. 23.
Shankman, P. (1976) *Migration and Underdevelopment: The Case of Western Samoa.* Boulder: Westview Press.
———. (1993) The Samoan exodus. In V. Lockwood et al. (eds.), *Contemporary Pacific Societies*, 156–170. Englewood Cliffs: Prentice Hall.
Shore, B. (1978) Introduction. In C. Macpherson, B. Shore and R. Franco (eds.), *New Neighbors . . . Islanders in Adaptation*, xiii–xiv. Santa Cruz: Center for South Pacific Studies.
Simpson, G. (1990) Wallerstein's world systems theory and the Cook Islands. *Pacific Studies* 14:73–94.
Small, C. (1997) *Voyages. From Tongan Villages to American Suburbs.* Ithaca: Cornell University Press.
Smith, R. (2004) Access to healthcare via telehealth: Experiences from the Pacific. *Perspectives on Global Development and Technology* 3:197–211.
So'o, A. (2001) Samoa. *The Contemporary Pacific* 13:246–255.
South Pacific Nurses Forum. (2002) *Record Of Meeting.* Vila: 11th South Pacific Nurses Forum.
Stewart, F. (2004) *Stories from Pacific Island Nurses.* Unpublished MEd thesis, Massey University, Palmerston North.
Taitai, T. (1999) *Health System Reform in the Western Pacific Region.* Manila: WHO.
Taylor, R. (1990) Problems of health administration in small states: Observations from the Pacific. In Y. Ghai (ed.), *Public Administration and Management in Small States. Pacific Experiences*, 60–114. Suva: Commonwealth Secretariat and USP.
———. (2008) History of public health in Pacific island countries. In M. Lewis and K. Macpherson (eds.), *Public Health in Asia and the Pacific*, 276–307. London: Routledge.
Taylor, R., D. Bampton and A. Lopez. (2005) Contemporary patterns of Pacific island mortality. *International Journal of Epidemiology* 18:634–646.
Tellei, J. and J. Renguul. (2003) Country Report on the Migration of Skilled Health Personnel in Pacific Island Countries: Palau. Unpublished paper presented to WHO Meeting on Migration of Skilled Health Personnel in Pacific Island Countries, Nadi.

Tenn, L., P. Sovaleni, R. Latu, A. Fotu and J. Smith. (1994) Getting the community involved in developing a PHC curriculum in Tonga. *International Nursing Review* 41 (5): 141–147.

Thaman, R. (2003) Consumerism, the media and malnutrition in the Pacific islands. *Pacific Health Dialog* 10 (1): 86–97.

Thomas, P. (2008) Indian nurses—seeking new shores. In J. Connell (ed.), *The International Migration of Health Workers*, 98–108. New York and London: Routledge.

Tokuda, A., G. Cernada and D. Kurahara. (2001) Health care in the freely associated states in Micronesia: Strategies beyond the compacts. *Pacific Heath Dialog* 8:207–212.

Tonga. (2000) *Tonga Nurses Association Country Paper.* Unpublished paper presented to 10th South Pacific Nurses Forum, Brisbane, October.

Tonga Ministry of Health. (2000) *Tonga's Health 2000*, Nuku'alofa: Ministry of Health.

Tsiaban, T. (2002) Role of the Nurse Practitioner in Vanuatu. Unpublished paper presented to 11th South Pacific Nurses Forum, Vila, August.

Tuqa, S. (1999) *Shortage of Local Doctors in the Civil Service* (mimeo). Suva: Ministry of Health.

United Nations. (1996) *Sustainable Human Development in Vanuatu.* Suva: United Nations.

———. (1998) *Sustainable Human Development in Palau.* Suva: United Nations.

United Nations Development Program (UNDP). (2005) *Republic of Vanuatu. Millennium Development Goals Report 2005.* Suva: UNDP.

———. (2007) *Human Development Report 2007/2008.* New York: UNDP.

Usher, K., G. Gray, J. Tollefson and L. Kerse. (2007) *Enhancing and Standardizing Regional Training Programmes in Nursing Mapping Exercise.* Townsville: James Cook University.

Usher, K. and D. Lindsay. (2003) The nurse practitioner role in Fiji: Results of an impact study. *Contemporary Nurse* 16 (1/2).

Utoikamanu, S. (2007) The Tongan economy 2007. *Pacific Economic Bulletin* 22 (3): 15–27.

Van Eyck, K. (2004) *Women and International Migration in the Health Sector.* Ferney-Voltaire: Public Services International.

Vanuatu. (2000) Vanuatu Nurses Association Country Report. Unpublished paper presented to 10th South Pacific Nurses Forum, Brisbane, October.

———. (2002) Vanuatu Nurses Association Country Report. Unpublished paper presented to 11th South Pacific Nurses Forum, Port Vila, August.

Vanuatu Ministry of Health. (2000) *2001 Human Resource Development Plan.* Port Vila: Ministry of Health.

Voigt-Graf, C. (2003) Fijian teachers on the move: Causes, implications and policies. *Asia-Pacific Viewpoint* 44:163–175.

Voigt-Graf, C., R. Iredale and S. Khoo. (2007) Teaching at home or overseas: Teacher migration from Fiji and the Cook Islands. *Asian and Pacific Migration Journal* 16:199–224.

Walsh, A.C. (1982) *Migration Urbanisation and Development in South Pacific Countries.* Bangkok: ESCAP.

Ward, M. (1971) *The Role of Investment in the Development of Fiji.* Cambridge: Cambridge University Press.

Ward, R.G. (1989) Earth's empty quarter? The Pacific islands in a Pacific century. *Geographical Journal* 155:235–246.

Ware, H. (2005) Demography, migration and conflict in the Pacific. *Journal of Peace Research* 42:435–454.

Wasuka, E. (2007) Cuban doctors to fill shortage. *Islands Business* 33 (5) May: 44–45.
Watson, W. (1964) Social mobility and social class in industrial communities. In M. Gluckman (ed.), *Closed Systems and Open Minds*, 129–157. Edinburgh: Oliver and Boyd.
Western, J. (1992) *A Passage to England. Barbadian Londoners Speak of Home*. London: UCL Press.
Wolfgramm, S. (1995) *Comments made by the National Health Development Committee on the Proposed Salary Structure and Interim Salary Revision for the Government Medical Practitioners of the Kingdom of Tonga* (mimeo). Nuku'alofa: Ministry of Health.
Workman, R., C. O'Meara, J. Craig, J. Nagel, E. Robbins and D. Ballendorf. (1981) *Island Voyagers in New Quests*. University of Guam: Micronesian Area Research Center.
World Bank. (1994) *Health Priorities in the World Bank's Pacific Member Countries*. Washington: World Bank.
———. (1998) *Samoa Health Sector Review. Meeting the Challenges of Development*. Washington: World Bank.
———. (2006) *At Home and Away*. Washington: World Bank.
———. (2007) *Opportunities to Improve Social Services. Human Development in the Pacific Islands*. Washington: World Bank.
World Health Organization (WHO). (2006a) *Country Health Information Profiles*. Manila: WHO.
———. (2006b) *Working Together For Health*. Geneva: WHO.
World Health Organization and Secretariat of the Pacific Community. (2006) *Pacific Code of Practice for Recruitment of Health Workers in the Pacific Region*. Suva: WHO.
Yeates, N. (2008) Here to stay? Migrant health workers in Ireland. In J. Connell (ed.), *The International Migration of Health Workers*, 61–75. New York and London: Routledge.

Index

K

L

M

N

O

P

For Product Safety Concerns and Information please contact our EU representative GPSR@taylorandfrancis.com
Taylor & Francis Verlag GmbH, Kaufingerstraße 24, 80331 München, Germany

www.ingramcontent.com/pod-product-compliance
Ingram Content Group UK Ltd.
Pitfield, Milton Keynes, MK11 3LW, UK
UKHW022119190926
475702UK00013B/1534
* 9 7 8 0 4 1 5 5 4 3 1 8 7 *